DEPARTMENT OF EDUCATION AND SCIENCE

Health Education in Schools

Her Majesty's Stationery Office

HE—A

ISBN 0 11 270456 5

CONTENTS

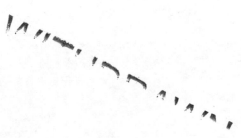

PREFACE

This book replaces Education Pamphlet No 49—Health and Education (1966) and A Handbook of Health Education (1968). It is not a comprehensive description of health education, but has been written to indicate recent developments and to point to some problems in health education in schools as they appear to a group of HM Inspectors and Medical Advisers to the Department of Education and Science.

The first four chapters are discussions of general principles. The remaining chapters deal in more detail with particular aspects of health education. Much of the subject matter is complex, emotive, and, in parts, speculative. Controversial topics and, therefore, value-judgements, can neither be ignored nor avoided. The book is issued in the hope that it will encourage further discussion and thought among parents, teachers, doctors, and young people alike. Nothing said is to be construed as implying government commitment to the provision of additional resources.

The references and suggestions for further reading are necessarily limited but include those which have been found especially helpful in the preparation of this book. A few (marked *) are more advanced than the others and demand some specialist knowledge.

HEALTH, PREVENTIVE MEDICINE AND HEALTH EDUCATION— SOME INTRODUCTORY IDEAS

Health is difficult to define. Some regard it as equivalent to freedom from disease. Others regard health as the harmonious interaction of the parts of the body, each of which is presumed to function efficiently. The World Health Organisation has adopted as a definition of health a state of complete physical, mental and social well-being. This implies that there are few, if any, aspects of life or of education which can be excluded from the ambit of health education.

Such a definition leads to so diffuse a view of the nature and role of health education in schools as to be of little practical significance. Health may more usefully be regarded as that combination of mental and physical states which gives rise to optimism and self-confidence; optimism and self-confidence rooted in an understanding of the working and limitations of body and mind, and of behaviour likely to minimise risk of mental and physical damage, avoiding the rashness of excessive indulgence on the one hand and the neurosis of hypochondria on the other. In this sense a person who is blind or mentally handicapped may be regarded as healthy, as and is entitled to contribute to and learn from health education as his more fortunate fellows.

Health, however defined, depends on a complex interaction between the environment, the genetic constitution of an individual, and behaviour by individuals and by groups.

Much of the preventive medicine in the past 2000 years has been directed to control of the environment, but as long ago as the codification of the Mosaic law the individual's need for personal hygiene has been recognised. The Romans understood the need for an abundant supply of clean water, efficient drainage and public conveniences, and devised the methods of civil engineering needed to provide them. They also observed a connection between marshy land and malaria, recognised contagion—venereal diseases have been understood by many generations to be contagious—isolated, and nearly eliminated, leprosy, and invented the military hospital. But although from ancient times the beliefs were widely held that infectious diseases originated from filth, excrement and other decomposing matter, and that the range of epidemics was related to areas of bad sanitation, by the beginning of the nineteenth century in England, cholera, typhoid, dysentery, typhus, smallpox and scarlet fever were still endemic, and sometimes epidemic, largely because of the growth of towns. The 'sanitarians', who believed that prevention consisted in getting rid of 'miasma' or 'effluvia', pressed their case, supported largely by studies of cholera epidemics early in the century. For the greater part of the nineteenth century they achieved more (through civil engineering) for the improvement of public health than doctors or scientists. They did not understand the aetiology of diseases or the factors which cause epidemics to wax and wane, but they hit on the right answers—which demanded communal action enforced by legislation—for combating them. Tuberculosis, the disease of dirt and over-crowding, began to decline in the 1830's. Cholera wholly disappeared in the 1860's, but the biological explanation of cholera was not understood until 1880.

Preventive medicine is not only a matter of sanitation, clean water, adequate diet and fresh air. Edward Jenner invented the technique of immunisation against specific diseases when he began vaccination against smallpox in 1796. This technique, which consists in stimulating the body to destroy its invaders, has resulted in the virtual elimination of smallpox, diptheria, poliomyelitis and tetanus throughout the Western World. Methods of killing pathogenic organisms outside the body were discovered in the middle of the nineteenth century—a discovery which, combined with the development of anaesthetics and the blood transfusion service, has made complex surgery possible. And, most significantly, the isolation of penicillin in 1928 began an era of biochemical research which has resulted in the synthesis of more and more substances capable of destroying germs inside the body without mobilising the body's own defences. This growth of chemotherapy, supported where appropriate by immunisation and vitally underpinned by hygiene (recent outbreaks of cholera and typhoid in various parts of the world serve as a reminder that we must never lose sight of the importance of sanitation and other measures of public health) has greatly changed the pattern of mortality in England and Wales, as in other countries, in the past 30 years.

Statistics of the causes of death began to be collected about 150 years ago. They are now published annually, with much other relevant data, by the Office of Population Censuses and Surveys. Table I, below, is a précis of these statistics for the years 1941, 1951, 1961 and 1971.

Table I

Death rates per million population (England and Wales), adapted from Table 8 in the Registrar General's Statistical Reviews of England and Wales.

(In these tables the 17 principal causes of death are sub-divided into approximately 200 causes based on an international classification amended in 1968.)

Classification	1941	1951	1961	1971
Population	42,000,000 (est)	43,815,000	46,197,000	48,815,000
Death rates per million	13,536	12,539	11,944	11,621
I Infective and parasitic diseases including	1,093	408	122	68
a. tuberculosis,	730	315	71	29
b. syphilis and other VD	80	35	10	3
II Neoplasms (cancers)	1,837	2,008	2,183	2,422
including trachea, bronchus and lung	253	487	492	630
III Endocrine, nutritional and metabolic diseases	95	179	120	137
IV Diseases of blood and blood forming organs	51	54	43	35
V Mental disorders		30	23	29
VI Diseases of nervous system and sense organs	206	141	128	127
VII Disease of circulatory system including	5,889*	6,051*	6,103*	6,014
a. cerebrovascular disease	1,247*	1,562*	1,668*	1,637
b. ischaemic heart disease, which includes			2,523*	2,932
acute myocardial infarction				
(coronary thrombosis)				(2,043)
VIII Diseases of respiratory system which include	1,807	1,863	1,610	1,527
a. influenza	177	361	153	14
b. pneumonia	687	536	635	811
c. bronchitis, emphysema and asthma	878	856	672	581
IX Diseases of digestive system	562	385	294	282
X Diseases of genito-urinary system	457	311	221	155
XIV Congenital anomalies	121	106	115	93
XVII Accidents, poisons and violence, including	1,119	451	505	463
a. traffic	165	103	141	142
b. falls	—	102	114	113
c. suicide	94	102	111	81

NB (1) Complications of pregnancy and childbirth (XI), Diseases of the skin (XII), Diseases of the musculoskeletal system (XIII), Certain causes of perinatal mortality, and symptoms, senility and ill-defined conditions (XVI) have been omitted for simplicity. These contributed a total rate of 153 in 1971, the most significant being senility (67) and rheumatism (33).

(2) Because of re-classification in 1968, resulting in a re-arrangement between categories VI and VII (before 1968 category VI included cerebrovascular disease, and the classification of heart disease in category VII was different) the figures marked* are approximate.

This extract is perhaps sufficiently detailed to indicate some of the difficulties in interpreting such data, difficulties which arise in part from precise definition of many causes of death and from the large number (about 1,000) of them listed in the tables. But enough is included to show a dramatic fall in deaths due to infective and parasitic diseases; a more modest fall in diseases of the digestive system and of the genito-urinary system; the persistent problem of accidents; and marked increases in fatal cancers (especially lung cancers), and in diseases of the circulatory system (especially forms of heart disease and coronary thrombosis).

The age at which death takes place is as important as its cause. Table II shows the age distribution of deaths (in raw figures) during 1971 from lung cancer, heart attack, pneumonia and road traffic accidents.

Table II
Ages of death in 1971 *due to four causes*

	0–9	10–19	20–29	30–39	40–49	50–59	60–69	70–79	80+
Lung cancer		3	42	170	1,498	5,630	12,126	9,068	
Heart attack		1	60	615	4,378	12,896	28,956	33,710	
Road accidents	765	1,246	1,226	524	559	707	900	867	460
Pneumonia	1,726	127	129	158	454	1,386	4,490	11,352	19,756

This shows in broad terms that road accidents, lung cancer and heart attack are of major significance among people below the age of retirement, while pneumonia is associated with deaths in infancy and, at the other end of the life span, remains the 'old man's friend'.

Table III summarises the expectation of life of men and women at various times in the twentieth century.

Table III
The expectation of life (England and Wales) at various ages, for the years 1901, 1931, 1951, 1971

	Males				Females			
Age	0	20	40	65	0	20	40	65
Date								
1901	48·5	43·0	27·0	10·8	52·4	45·8	29·4	12·0
1931	58·7	46·8	29·6	11·3	62·9	49·9	32·6	13·1
1951	65·8	49·1	30·5	11·2	70.9	53·5	34·7	13·8
1971	69·0	51·1	32·0	12·2	75·3	56·9	37·6	16·1

NB   The expectation of life at a particular age is the average number of years which a population could be expected to survive beyond that age, if the population continued to have the mortality rates in that particular calendar year. At birth it is the expected average survival period of the population born in that year, calculated from the mortality rates in each age group of the whole population that year, so a (current) life table is built up which gives a useful summary of mortality, on the arbitrary assumption that the population will continue to experience the mortality rates of the given year throughout life.

Although the decline in tuberculosis, typhus, typhoid, cholera, dysentery and smallpox in the second half of the nineteenth century obviously increased expectation of life at birth the greatest single contribution to the improvements in death rates was the fall in infant mortality, which came later in the cycle of change. This began to fall rapidly from about 150 per 1,000 live births at the end of the last century, and is now (1961–70) about 20 deaths under 1 year per 1,000 live births.

Table IV, taken from the Registrar General's *Statistical reviews*, summarises the number of cases of the principal notifiable infectious diseases at 10 year intervals during the past 30 years. These are of course not necessarily fatal.

Table IV
Notifications of infectious diseases in England and Wales

	1941	1951	1961	1971
Typhoid	1,034	206	97	131
Paratyphoid fever	3,621	1,095	254	91
Cholera	0	0	0	3
Acute meningitis	9,886	1,390	651	1,881
Scarlet fever	95,551	48,744	19,990	12,490
Whooping cough	173,249	169,441	24,470	16,846
Diptheria	49,432	664	52	17
Dysentery	6,389	28,590	20,418	10,680
Smallpox	0	0	1	1
Measles	407,949	616,192	763,531	135,241
Acute poliomyelitis	—	1,614	876	7
Food poisoning	—	5,799	7,842	6,727

Data on the causes and effects of illness in the adult population are neither easy to obtain not to interpret. Table V below gives at least some clues about the extent of ill-health in the adult population.

Table V
The 12 main causes of illness in 1968 (the latest year for which data are available), estimated by a 5 per cent sample of claimants for sickness benefit under the National Insurance Acts, measured in millions of days of absence from work, abstracted from Table 11.3 in the *Digest of health statistics for England and Wales*, Department of Health and Social Security, 1971, where 26 classes of illness are listed.

	(*million*)
Total number of days illness	327·6
Bronchitis	38·6
Symptoms, senility, and ill defined conditions (ie not feeling well)	31·3
Mental, psychoneurotic and personality disorders	30·7
Accidents, poisonings and violence	27·0
Diseases of the digestive system	26·1

Diseases of the respiratory system (except bronchitis)   25·4
Arthritis and rheumatism (except rheumatic fever)   23·1
Diseases of the circulatory system, except arteriosclerotic
   and degenerative heart diseases   20·3
Arteriosclerotic and degenerative heart diseases   18·1
Influenza   15·5
Inflammatory and other diseases of the nervous system   15·5
Diseases of bones and other organs of movement   8·5
(The remaining 14 causes combined   37)

Women are probably under-represented in these statistics because many married women have chosen not to be insured for sickness benefit.

These data present a disturbing picture of illness, despite advances in public health and in the application of science to medicine. The great loss of time and the unhappiness implied as a consequence of respiratory diseases, mental illness, accidents, diseases of the digestive system, arthritis and rheumatism and ill-defined states of 'not feeling well' give no grounds for complacency. They also remind us that illness as well as early death is a target for preventive medicine, and that the remarkable expansion of the pharmacopoeia in the past 20 years has not conquered illness although it has greatly improved treatment.

The mortality tables give reasonable evidence that the so called 'stress diseases', or 'diseases of civilisation', are replacing infectious and contagious diseases as causes of death. Because of the success of good sanitation, improved nutrition, immunisation, chemotherapy and more sophisticated surgical techniques, many now survive infections, eventually to die of cancer and ischaemic heart disease, but may live long enough to spend a period in a geriatric hospital. This change of emphasis in no way undermines the traditional foundation of health education in hygiene—it adds other important factors. Today a man may greatly reduce the risk of his death by lung cancer by his own choice whereas even 50 years ago he could not reduce the risk of his death from tuberculosis unless supporting action was taken by the community, enforced by law.

Except for the figures for death from lung cancer, accidents and venereal diseases (nowadays often called sexually transmitted diseases to obscure their association with venery) the tables given above do not directly present evidence of death and illness caused by habits, or individual behaviour. Such growing hazards include alcoholism and the direct and indirect consequences of excessive drinking (although no doubt many a hangover is disguised under more reputable labels in table V); unwanted pregnancy and, sometimes, abortion; venereal diseases; 'bad trips' from LSD; obesity; and 'stress' illnesses as well as mental breakdown associated with obsessive overwork or failure to co-operate harmoniously with other people. All of these sources of ill health are based on irrational or inconsiderate behaviour by individuals, but they are rarely a consequence of individual action alone, so that sociology (a study of the influence of the group) as well as psychology is involved. As many, if not all, actions leading to such illness affect, and often show lack of regard for, other people, and as some may offend the religious beliefs of a substantial proportion of the population, questions of morality and of religion are not far below the surface when nowadays preventive medicine in its broadest sense is discussed.

Except perhaps in part for the entry under congenital abnormalities in Table I the data above give little direct indication of the effect of genetic factors on diseases transmitted from generation to generation, or on variations of human development; or variation in resistance or susceptibility to a wide range of diseases; or on aspects of behaviour, including the ability to learn, which are in part genetically determined. The broad concept of human variation is fundamental to understanding of any epidemiological arguments and to a great deal of health education.

Epidemiology, the study of disease patterns and of the factors in the environment and in behaviour which are related to the incidence and spread of disease, is dependent on medical statistics, which, as has already been stated, began to be collected in England and Wales about 150 years ago. In principle such studies are simple matters of relating cause and effect, as, for example, the Romans' association of marshy land with malaria. In practice they are usually complex, because of the very large number of factors involved and because some effects may be masked by others. There is a well-known observation by Dr John Snow in 1854 that those who drew water from the Broad Street pump had a greater risk of dying from cholera than those who used an adjacent supply of pure water from Thames Ditton. This led him to deduce that cholera was 'caused' by polluted water (an argument which because of human variation rested on what he called 'statistical observations and relationships'). The story is an early example of successful epidemiology —successful before the germ theory of cholera was understood. A recent example is that the argument establishing a causal connection between cigarette smoking and lung cancer, also rooted in 'statistical observations and relationships', was set out before the biological mechanism by which cigarette smoke may trigger the formation of carcinomas was fully understood. Such studies are gaining in importance and in practicability because of rapid progress in data-handling techniques, the growth of computer science, and international co-operation in the collection of data. Their role in preventive medicine is related, not only to studying 'causes' of epidemics but to projecting the present trends into future patterns of disease.

The growth of data-handling techniques has increased the possibility of screening, a process which can lead to the detection of physiological or anatomical abnormalities before a disease in its usual form can be diagnosed. These techniques have economic implications, which need not be discussed here, and are dependent for their success on a degree of understanding of their purpose by the public. They are potentially a growing element in preventive medicine. The service known until 1 April 1974 as the School Health Service was largely engaged in another important aspect of screening.

To summarise, preventive medicine is based on hygiene, sanitation and nutrition; on immunisation; on epidemiology; and screening. The state of the art, at least in the Western world, presents a health spectrum of which Professor L S Levin of Yale University said in a lecture to the Society for Health Education in 1973:

' we see a shift in disease patterns from acute infectious diseases to chronic disease; a conceptual shift from disease cure to health maintenance; and a shift in people's expectations towards greater control of their own lives . . . The goal is to strengthen individual health behaviours . . .'.

All of the elements of preventive medicine demand individual knowledge and judgement, so that education—health education as it is called—is itself an element of preventive medicine of growing importance and increasing complexity. Clearly not all health education, however defined, is directly the responsibility of schools. The foundations of behaviour and of knowledge in which health education is rooted are best laid in the home.

These changes in medicine have been accompanied by equally significant changes in schools of all kinds since 1944. Boys and girls are now more often encouraged to investigate for themselves, to examine the bases of established conventions, to handle data and to draw their own conclusions from them. The study of child development has advanced, and the great variations in the time and rate of physical, emotional and intellectual growth are increasingly understood by teachers. The curriculum has widened. In secondary schools preoccupation with external examinations has grown and with it the danger that that which cannot be examined, such as some aspects of health education, is not worth consideration by the intellectually more gifted. The content of the curriculum is being challenged and revised not only by individual teachers but by groups of teachers and others working in curriculum development groups sponsored, in the first instance, by the Nuffield Foundation and the Schools Council, and now also by the Health Education Council. These reformers, whatever their disciplines, seek on the one hand to encourage boys and girls to think for themselves and on the other hand to present knowledge which may be seen by them to be relevant in their lives. At the same time relationships between pupils in secondary schools and teachers have tended to become less formal and many matters which were taboo even 10 years ago may now be discussed (and often are) with propriety in school as elsewhere. Boys and girls show less patience than their parents with institutional forms of control but perhaps more readily accept social responsibilities such as care for the aged or deprived. Their freedom in one sense has grown, possibly because more money is available to many of them, but their freedom in another sense is restricted by demands for academic success imposed on more and more of them by the increasing complexity and competitive-ness of entry requirements for many jobs and for courses in further education.

Health education is capable of many definitions. For the purposes of this pamphlet a pragmatic view will be adopted. Health education will be regarded as that part of education—the responsibility of parents, the schools, and indeed the whole community—which will help boys and girls as they grow up to minimise the risks of diseases and injuries resulting wholly or in part from ignorance, habits and ways of living, and give them a basis of understanding of the functions of the com-munity health services so that they may be able to use them intelligently and efficiently and play their parts in reaching wise decisions on their evolution as patterns of illness change.

About a hundred years ago the headmaster of Winchester College commented on the science taught in his school:

'. . . every man of liberal education is the better for not being ignorant of anything, but compared with other things a scientific fact is a fact which pro-duces nothing in a boy's mind. It is simply a barren fact which he remembers or does not remember for a time and after a few years becomes confused with other facts and is forgotten. It leads to nothing. It does not germinate, it is a perfectly unfruitful fact . . . I think except on the part of those who have a taste for the physical sciences and intend to pursue them as amateurs or professionals, such instruction is worthless as education.'

No headmaster today would so denigrate the contribution of science to education, because ways have evolved of presenting science not as a series of unfruitful and unrelated facts, but as a rich source of ideas based on facts; ideas which germinate and are capable of stretching the minds of even the most gifted.

There are encouraging signs that health education is developing from a set of facts and admonitions into studies which demand the exercise of judgement based on knowledge derived from several disciplines, and on the assessment of probabilities. Professor Levin, in the course of the lecture referred to earlier, put these ideas forcibly when he said:

'. . . for years school health education (in the United States) used the "tell them the facts" approach. It was found, however, that this had very limited effect on children's health behaviour. As the problem was examined from the standpoint of learning theory and behaviour change, it became clear that much more was involved than merely creating an awareness of health, disease, and necessary protective action. It was also found necessary to involve the child in an analytic, testing and decision-making process; analytic in the sense of sorting out evidence, interpreting that evidence, making judgements of saliency, weighing merits of various solutions, and making a decision with regard to health behaviour both at the individual and social levels. This is a more time-consuming approach. It is also more satisfying to both child and teacher. It avoids homogenised, stereotyped solutions with low credibility. It has the many benefits inherent in participating in a scientific enterprise—emphasising a problem solving technique which will outlast by many years the five year half-life of many health facts. In America we are a long way from universal or even major application of such methods even though they are thoroughly rational in terms of both learning theory and health behaviour change . . .'.

And so are we. The main purpose of this pamphlet is to encourage such approaches to health education without claiming an unrealistic share of the total activities of schools.

References

Statistical reviews for England and Wales, Registrar General, Office of Population Censuses and Surveys, HMSO, yearly.

Health education, Report of the Cohen Committee (Ministry of Health, HMSO, 1964.

'Expectation of Life', *Sociology in medicine* pp 26–31 in M W Susser and W Watson, OUP, 1971.

Further reading

Science and public health (Block 5, unit 10), R G Hodgkinson, Open University Press, 1973.

'The Changing Patterns of Disease', Part 4 in *A natural history of man,* J K Brierley, Heinemann, 1970.

*'Economy, Population and Health' (Pt. 1) and *'Social Class and Disorders of Health', (Pt. 4, in *Sociology in medicine,* M W Susser and W Watson, OUP, 1971.

*Chapter 15, on screening, in *Data handling in epidemiology,* W W Holland (Ed.), OUP, 1970.

'The Community's Health', Ch. 4 in *A textbook of health education* (Second edition), A J Dalzell Ward, Tavistock Publications, 1974.

2

HEALTH SERVICES AND HEALTH EDUCATION

At the beginning of this century, when medical opinion had been alerted by the poor physical condition of many young men who had been rejected by the Army for service in the Boer War, an interdepartmental committee recommended that the medical inspection of school children should be a statutory duty of local education authorities. This duty was imposed on authorities by the Education Act of 1907, when the Board of Education issued a circular which stated that school medical inspections should be done

'with a view to adapting and modifying the system of education to the needs and capabilities of the child, securing the early detection of unsuspected defects, checking incipient maladies at their outset, and furnishing the facts that will guide Education Authorities in relation to physical and mental development during school life.'

The clear intention from the beginning was that the service should be preventive rather than curative, but disease was soon seen to be so prevalent among school children that a treatment service had to be provided. Malnutrition, rickets, and a variety of infestations were the commonest medical problems. Handicapping eye and ear diseases and crippling physical difficulties as a consequence of osteomyelitis, rheumatic fever and poliomyelitis pointed to the need not only for medical treatment but for special educational facilities:

'Successive education enactments established the duty of local authorities to provide for the medical inspection of pupils in schools they maintain, and the Education Act 1944 extended this duty to securing the provision of free medical treatment. Parents are invited and encouraged to attend school medical inspections.'

As the health of school children improved, treatment by the School Medical Service decreased, until in 1946 the formation of the National Health Service largely relieved the service of this obligation so that it was able to concentrate on early diagnosis and referral.

In the period from 1946 until 31 March 1974 the School Health Service became highly organised to monitor the health of school children (see Chapter 1). Preventive medicine was practised using regular routine medical examinations, screening techniques and immunisation procedures against the more dangerous of the infectious diseases. School doctors became more involved in the assessment of physically and mentally handicapped children and careful routine medical examinations were made to detect any brain damage (however slight) that could affect a child's ability to benefit from his schooling. These developments gradually led to better liaison between school doctors, parents, teachers and psychologists. In the same period health visitors and school nurses, as well as maintaining their regular hygiene inspections, undertook routine testing of sight and colour vision, and, in some areas, of hearing, and ensured that individual immunisation schedules were up to date. In recent years an increasing number of large secondary schools have appointed qualified nurses to their staffs. The number of speech therapists, audiometricians and physiotherapists working in the school medical service rose substantially. Doctors inspected school premises to ensure that ventilation, heating and lighting were adequate and some of them became involved in health education in the classroom. When free milk was no longer available to primary school children over seven, the school doctor was empowered to issue a certificate for a supply of free milk for such children in primary schools whose physical condition warranted it.

Up to 1 April 1974, in all but two local authorities, School Health and Maternal and Child Welfare were administered by a doctor with the joint appointment of Medical Officer of Health and Principal School Medical Officer, and were staffed by doctors working in both fields. So the more serious handicaps were picked up before the children concerned were five years old and the special educational provisions allowed them to be placed in suitable teaching establishments from as early an age as two years. Children discovered to be handicapped were mainly found to have sensory disorders of vision or hearing or were mentally retarded.

The identification of some children who needed help took place later as their problems did not become apparent until they had been in school for some time. This was particularly true for behavioural difficulties and emotional problems. The peak age for referrals for such difficulties was between eight and ten years. Placement in a school for the educationally subnormal almost invariably depended on a medical opinion given by a doctor who was specially qualified to do so, but assessment by an educational psychologist and a teacher acting together was becoming increasingly common.

During this period the Department of Education and Science published biennially *The health of the school child*, a mine of information to teachers and others interested in the changes and improvements of the health, including dental health, of generations of children. The report published in 1972 includes the statement that less than one per cent of school entrants were considered to be in unsatisfactory health. This is a remarkable tribute to a quiet revolution in this century and especially to the work of Maternal and Child Welfare Services, whose health visitors contributed greatly to the health education of parents, and thus of children, and so helped to provide an essential foundation on which the schools could build.

On 1 April 1974 all the local authority medical services, including the School Medical Service, were incorporated into the National Health Service and came under the administration of the Department of Health and Social Security in England, and the Welsh Office in Wales. The arrangements are described in National Health Service Re-organisation Circular HRC (74)5 issued by the Department of Health and Social Security, and in WHRC (74)7 issued by the Welsh Office. These documents detail the responsibilities of medical, dental and nursing staff to the Child Health Service and include the following reference to health education in schools:

Health education within the school curriculum is the responsibility of local education authorities and schools. There is, however, an important continuing role for school health services' staff in participating with teaching staff in the planning and presentation of health education programmes, which may involve parents as well as pupils, and in advising pupils and their parents individually. This is a matter for close liaison between area health authorities and local education authorities.'

The essential change brought about by the National Health Service Re-organisation Act 1973 is that the school health service has been replaced by a child health service controlled at Area Health Authority level by an Area Specialist in Community Medicine (Child Health), with an Area Dental Officer and an Area Nursing Officer (Child Health). The objective was to establish a comprehensive range of integrated health services for children from birth until they leave school. This has been done by co-ordinating the activities of general medical and dental practitioners, the hospital and specialist services, the medical and dental inspection and treatment of school children, and local authority health services for the pre-school child. School medical and dental officers have been transferred to Area Health Authorities which have the following major responsibilities to local education authorities:

a. to ensure that pupils are in the best health possible so as to benefit fully from attendance at school;
b. to ensure that medical and other necessary health service staff are available to enable local education authorities to continue to discharge their responsibilities under the Education Act 1944 (sections 33 and 34) to pupils requiring special educational treatment; and
c. to provide a medical advisory service to local education authorities, to teachers and parents to help them in providing education according to the age, aptitude and ability of every child.

Schools are still visited by a doctor and medical examinations of children take place in schools. The annual inspection of large numbers of children is being replaced by more frequent visits by the doctor to the school. Fewer children are examined at any one visit but there is more time for investigation into the medical and social problems of an individual child in his class, school and home and for subsequent discussion with headmasters and headmistresses, teachers and parents. The head of a school should be able to seek medical advice on a child whenever necessary. These changes imply a closer professional working relationship between teachers and doctors, and the prospect that teachers may learn more of the medical aspects of health education from doctors who in their turn will increasingly come to appreciate, as many do, that teaching is slow, subtle and sometimes difficult.

Another National Health Service Re-organisation Circular (HRC (74)27) issued by the Department of Health and Social Security and WHRC (74)22 from the Welsh Office describe the functions of health authorities, local authorities and the Health Education Council in relation to health education, and the effect in this field of the re-organisation of the National Health Service and of local government. This circular refers specifically to health education in schools and colleges in the following terms:

'Health education work in schools varies but, whether as a recognisable study in its own right or as part of the teaching in many subject areas, or within the pastoral life of the school, it is growing in importance. Colleges of education offer some instruction in its elements and college tutors responsible for this work are concerned with the development of new methods of presentation. Health education advice may also be provided by higher and further education establishments for their students. There is much scope for collaboration on health education between area health authorities, local education authorities and other educational bodies in their areas. As well as health education officers, doctors, dentists, health visitors, school nurses, public health inspectors and chiropodists already contribute to health education work in schools, and this should continue. Area health authorities should be prepared to co-operate with local education authorities, education establishments, teachers and parents associations in assisting in identifying health education needs, and by providing speakers, materials, information and advice on health education matters. They should also be prepared to help local education authorities in the in-service training of teachers in health education. Area health authorities will no doubt find the experience of the education service of value in considering ways of effectively communicating with young people on health education topics. Area health authorities should aim to establish close working relationships with all appropriate local education interests as soon as possible.'

This circular also points out that an area medical officer will be responsible to his area health authority for drawing up health education programmes as part of his wider role in developing preventive health services, thus officially recognising health education for the whole community as part of preventive medicine. Area medical officers will be advised by other professional colleagues including area nursing officers and area health education officers. Area health education officers, who will normally be directly accountable to area medical officers, have executive responsibility for all health education work except for what is taught in schools, which of course remains the responsibility of headmasters and headmistresses, who are accountable to their governing bodies and, in the maintained sector, to the local education authority.

Health education officers, the majority of whom trained initially as health visitors, teachers, or public health inspectors, have rapidly increased in numbers since the Cohen Committee on Health Education reported in 1964 (see references). They are appointed to area health authorities. They are responsible for encouraging health education in all age groups, and although their rights do not extend to uninvited entry to schools they are available to teachers for advice, for up-to-date information, for access to resources, and for help with courses for teachers.

The increasing number of appointments of health education officers has been accompanied by a smaller rise in the number of local education authority advisers with responsibility for health education, often as part of wider responsibilities. The health education advisers are able to be in close contact with medical thought and opinion and also to discuss their professional concerns with colleagues whose interests are primarily in education. Health education officers see health education in schools in relation to a wider field of health education while the advisers see it in relation to the total activities of schools. So these officials, responsible to different branches of the public service, are not rivals; on the contrary they are especially well placed to complement one another.

The Cohen Committee included among its recommendations:

'The Government should establish a strong Central Board in England and Wales which would promote a climate of opinion generally favourable to health education, develop "blanket" programmes of education on selected priority subjects, securing support from all possible national sources, commercial and voluntary as well as medical and assist local authorities and other agencies in the conduct of programmes locally. It would foster the training of specialist health educators, promote the training in health education of doctors, nurses, teachers and dentists; and evaluate the results achieved by health education.'

The Health Education Council was established by the government in 1968 and is concerned with the planning and promotion of health education at national level in England, Wales and Northern Ireland. The Council is an independent body financed from the Exchequer. All the members are appointed by the Secretary of State for Social Services, including some nominated by the Secretaries of State for Education and Science, for Wales, and for Northern Ireland.

The work of the Council of which many people will be especially aware is its publicity. This includes press coverage and reference to health education topics in several well-known programmes on national and regional television and radio networks. Some campaigns, such as those on smoking and pregnancy, and on family planning, have attracted widespread attention and comment. Less spectacular aspects of its work are perhaps of greater interest and concern to teachers engaged in health education and are not so widely known. These include the reviewing of relevant medical, epidemiological, sociological and psychological information and, when necessary, sponsoring research designed to obtain such information to help the Council to determine its priorities and to increase the effectiveness of its campaigns as well as the many activities of its education and training division.

The Council's main functions are summarised in an appendix to DHSS Circular HRC (74)27 and WHRC (74)22 (Welsh Office). Those responsibilities most directly related to the work of teachers include

acting as a national centre of expertise and knowledge in all aspects of health education;

encouraging and promoting training in health education work;

co-operating with local education authorities, educational establishments and the Schools Council in the development of health education in schools, colleges and polytechnics;

maintaining contact with national voluntary bodies engaged in particular aspects of health education work, and

publishing material of interest and value to those engaged in health education.

The Council has established at its headquarters in London an extensive library and a resources centre open to teachers for the examination of films, tapes etc; has encouraged the setting up of advanced diploma courses in polytechnics for teachers and health education officers, and part-time courses in colleges of further education for those, such as health visitors, whose work includes health education; has supported the Schools Council in a curriculum development project and has sponsored another for which it is alone responsible. The Council's officials take their places in the committees of many national societies and voluntary bodies. These activities are conveniently summarised from time to time in the Council's free bulletin *Health education news for teachers* which is proving a valuable source of information not only about the work of the Council and other bodies but also about experiments by teachers from different parts of the country, and thus serves as a forum for the exchange of ideas and experience.

The matters so far referred to in this chapter have been included primarily as information for teachers, but some at least of them are the concern of parents if they are to understand the provisions made for the medical care of children and the ways in which these may gradually be improved. It was pointed out in Chapter 1 that knowledge of the purpose of the health service is a necessary part of health education to enable boys and girls to use the service sensibly and, when they grow up, to understand why changing circumstances will impose changes on the service and to play their role in helping to ensure that wise decisions on its evolution are made. Examples of changes since the National Health Service was set up are: the average length of stay in hospitals by in-patients is now about half what it was twenty years ago; the incidence of accidents needing hospital treatment has nearly doubled; and hospital medical staff has increased by about a quarter while the number of family doctors has remained virtually unchanged. From 1955 to 1968 there was a 30 per cent increase in absence from work for sickness, due mainly to less serious complaints.

When the national health service was planned, sickness was usually the result of infection or accident, often successfully cured, or a deteriorating chronic condition for which little could be done. Today, as we have implied in Chapter 1, health, like illness, is increasingly difficult to define. Health, like illness, depends increasingly on personal decision. The subjective judgement of an individual often decides whether he is well or sick. This last point is illustrated in Table VI.

Table VI
Attitude to jobs of men with various spells of sickness absence
(P J Taylor—see references)

Absence group	Enjoy job percentage	Indifferent to job percentage	Dislike job percentage
Frequently sick	46	36	18
Control group:	80	16	4
(Matched with frequently sick)			
Long term sickness	74	20	6
Never off sick	96	2	2
Percentage of all men	72	20	8
Number of men	142	37	15

In addition, as has been stated in a recent paper from the Office of Health Economics (see references)

'The borderline between health and sickness has been advancing in a new direction. Obesity, alcoholism, depression, sexual deviations and even strained family relationships are increasingly regarded as diseases justifying treatment . . . With these sorts of disorders the problem of definition becomes almost insuperable. Few people live perfectly balanced and adjusted lives and it would be possible to identify for everyone some abnormal or eccentric attitudes or patterns of behaviour . . .'

Today there is no sharp demarcation, but a continuous gradation between health and sickness; we all have almost unlimited scope for regarding ourselves as sick. Conditions which were regarded as chronic and even hopeless in the thirties may be cured, or at least ameliorated, so the expectation and demand of everyone for treatment or alleviation of distress have risen greatly. Illnesses may be so stabilised by drugs that they no longer preclude a healthy life provided that some limitations, such as the inability of a diabetic to qualify as an airline pilot, are accepted. Illness may soon come to be regarded as a combination of conditions, often temporary, which necessitates withdrawal from society. The healthier the population becomes the more sickness is reported, and the more insistent becomes the demand for treatment. On the other hand there is evidence that many people with significant medical abnormalities receive no treatment because they do not recognise their need, and give their doctors no chance of detecting them.

These are some of the changes in society and in medicine which impose changes on the health service. Their discussion is a neglected part of health education.

References

Health of the school child, DES, HMSO, Biennial until issue for 1971/2, now ceased publication.

Health education 'Personal factors connected with sickness absence; a study of 194 men with contrasting sickness absence experience in a refinery situation, in Report of the Cohen Committee, HMSO, 1964.

British journal of industrial medicine vol. 25, pt. 2, pp. 106–118, P J Taylor, British Medical Association, April, 1968.

Reorganisation Circulars HRC (74)5 and (74) 27, DHSS, HMSO, 1974.

Bulletins for Teachers, Health Education Council, HEC, various.

Newsletters, Health Education Council, HEC, various.

Further reading

'The National Health Service' (Pt. 3, sec. 1) 'Prospects in Health'** (Pt. 3, sec. 3) in *Decision making in Britain* Block V—Health, Open University Press, 1972.

Note** Reprint of Office of Health Economics **Paper 37, 1971.**

'The School Health Service', Ch. 14 in *A textbook of health education*, Dr A J Dalzell-Ward, Tavistock Publications, 1974.

3

BIOLOGY AND HEALTH EDUCATION IN SCHOOLS

Biology is a necessary but not a sufficient basis for health education.

We shall begin by considering a few of the biological ideas implied in the statement in Chapter 1 that health depends on an interaction between the environment, the genetic constitution of the individual, and the behaviour of individuals and of groups.

The environment is obviously partly describable in biological terms because it includes a vast range of living organisms. Ecology, the study of living things in relation to their surroundings, including other living things, is a very important branch of modern biology. Boys and girls need gradually to understand that they live in a continuously changing state of equilibrium with many plants and animals which not only compete with them for space and food, but supply them with food and maintain an atmosphere which they can breathe. They need, too, to appreciate the effects on this equilibrium when a deliberate effort is made to shift it to their immediate advantage as, for example, by the use of insecticides. Chapter 6 is concerned with one aspect of these complex interactions—the spread, control, and sometimes the elimination, of infectious diseases caused and propagated by many different minute organisms.

Genetics is at the heart of biology. It is difficult to exaggerate the significance of inherited characteristics to individual health because of the genetic factor in determining resistance to diseases. The best way for a man to give himself a prospect of good health would be for him to choose his parents wisely!

Behaviour is the field in which the limitations of biology, as of all natural science, are exposed. For example, at the appropriate level of biology teaching it is possible to explain how the nerves, hormones, and a variety of organic systems interact to develop the stages of the stress reaction, or the physiological response of the body to pain, heat and danger. But this knowledge by itself tells no one how to cope with those who are under stress, or how to ameliorate the stress to which people may be subject. A moment's consideration of the range of skill and knowledge needed to enable anyone to do this demonstrates that biological science alone is not enough.

In many primary schools children are encouraged to observe and to care for plants and animals. They talk about them and build up an appropriate vocabulary. They talk about themselves and learn the names and usually the purposes of parts of their bodies. They learn that plants and animals provide food. This is the beginning of an understanding of the interdependence of man and other living things: it can also be the beginning of the all-important understanding of nutrition, of what is good to eat, and why. By keeping animals such as gerbils or hamsters in school, as well as by helping to look after family pets, children learn what animals need: warmth, food, water, a place to sleep and a place to play. These needs are not so different, except for one vital omission, from their own, as they may realise for themselves. They learn, too, to handle animals. This emphasises the teaching of simple hygiene. It is not enough to train children to wash their hands after handling animals, after visiting the lavatory, and before meals. They need to know why they must do so. This is the beginning of learning about infection and the control of diseases, and the beginning of the idea of responsibility for one's own health and that of others.

In the last century human anatomy and physiology were taught in schools but with no reference to reproduction and sex. It would be ironic if today we taught about reproduction and sex with no reference to other bodily functions. Children are often interested in their bodies and a simple biological approach, provided that it is not so simplified that it is misleading, is appropriate in the junior school. Such teaching may encourage the formation of responsible attitudes to the care and maintenance of the body.

Genetics, although it would not be so described to young children, introduces the idea of variation and thus the possibility of discussion of what is meant by normal. At a very simple level, by measuring an index of body size such as the dimensions of their hands boys and girls can arrive at the normal distribution curve and the notion of acceptable limits of variation before anyone is considered to be unusual, and thus come to the idea that every society or group within society has its view of what is acceptable in its members.

Children, too, may well ask why they grow ('because they eat' is not a satisfactory answer), why some grow faster than others, and why they eventually stop growing after going through a series of changes. At a very early stage children begin to classify. When they recognise the essential similarities between an Alsatian and a Pekinese—whose differences are much greater than the differences among boys or girls—they have grasped another important idea. When they realise that they more closely resemble their brothers and sisters and their parents than other people, and that every human being is different from every other, they are beginning to grasp another important principle.

Enough has been touched on to illustrate some of the ways in which children acquire biological ideas and the beginnings of health education from an early age. In secondary schools, when many but by no means all boys and girls start a more systematic study of biology, the problem for health education is to extend the discussion to consideration of kinds of behaviour and their effects. At times it is necessary for the teacher only to make explicit the implications for health of a topic, such as the understanding of a physiological system. At other times it may be more useful deliberately to slant the teaching of biology towards health maintenance. For example, in a study of body temperature the biologist would consider the temperature of a variety of organisms, including invertebrates as well as vertebrates. Cold-blooded and warm-blooded animals would be observed and such questions as the following might be raised: What is the significance for the organism of being cold- or warm-blooded? What is the significance for man of a (nearly) constant high temperature? How is this temperature regulated? What are the functions of the hypothalamus, of subcutaneous fat, and of sweating? What are the effects of metabolic rate? These questions are all interesting and appropriate but by themselves they do not necessarily make boys and girls capable of intelligent behaviour when they have a high temperature, because they find it difficult to translate such knowledge into practical action. But the teacher may help them to make such a translation by asking such further questions as: What are normal temperatures? Does your temperature change after a cold drink, or throughout the day, or with changes in the temperature and humidity of the air? What is your body telling you by raising its temperature? Ought you to try and get it down? Is it sensible to have a cold bath to bring the temperature down? Or to take aspirins? Are there any dangers?

This rather trivial example is within the experience of every child and the transition to health education is simple. Some teachers may prefer to begin with the observable facts of variations in human temperature and lead back to an understanding of the biological ideas. In the stress reaction mentioned earlier the transition is much more difficult.

A broad physiological view of man may help older boys and girls to respect the complexity, organisation and working of body and mind, and give them confidence in the ability of the body to adapt and to heal itself. This view presents the body as constructed of millions of intricate parts, each designed for a particular job. Specialised cells are organised into systems (eg the central nervous system) which together carry out essential life-support activities on behalf of the whole body. For example, the lungs control the oxygen intake and the kidneys control the water-balance. The major systems are linked together by nerves and circulatory fluids so that the rate of operation of each system can be changed when necessary. The circulating fluids have a chemical composition which varies within narrow limits: any change in the level of any ingredient is detected by monitoring systems and the appropriate regulatory action is taken. Minute changes in concentration can be detected and in some instances have dramatic effects on the action of a system, as when the hormone oxytocin causes the womb to contract and expel the foetus. Changes in the internal fluids are brought about by changes in the activity of man or by changes in his environment: in a stressful situation fuel is liberated and diverted to organs vital for escape or survival. Most of these activities which co-ordinate the diverse functions of the body or adapt its rate of working to the environmental demand are carried out automatically. The body is self-repairing and to a large extent self-replacing, and the female body is capable of reproduction with initial help from the male. Such an intricate self-maintaining organism is not to be tampered with lightly by those in search of kicks or by those who at the least sign of discomfort demand drugs to cure all ills.

A more difficult part of health education is to strengthen attitudes which increase the probability of behaviour likely to lessen the long-term risks of illnesses which to boys and girls are in the distant and unimagined future. One example showing how elementary biology may help is in possible extensions to teaching about the closely interrelated topics of respiration, the circulation of the blood, and nutrition—topics difficult to understand if studied in isolation.

Diseases of the circulatory and of the respiratory systems, including lung cancer, nowadays account for nearly half the deaths (and for a substantial proportion of ill health) among the middle aged and elderly who live in industrial countries. The efficiency of the gas exchange mechanism of the lungs is clearly related to their effective surface area, so that if the usable surface is reduced by damage or destruction more work will be demanded of the heart to collect and deliver a given volume of oxygen needed for the working of every muscle including the heart muscle. It is almost obvious that temporary or permanent damage to the circulatory system is probable if the efficiency of the gas exchange mechanism of the lungs is impaired by hostile micro-organisms or by substances such as asbestos dust, sulphur dioxide, and tobacco smoke, all of which are known to be capable of inflicting irreparable (and ultimately fatal) damage if they are in contact with working surfaces of the lungs for prolonged periods.

Diseases of the circulation, often called diseases of the blood vessels, may take the form either of disease of the arteries or of disease of the heart itself. Degenerative diseases of the arteries, which may begin in middle age, are known collectively as arterio-sclerosis.

Plaques of atheroma (products of fat metabolism) may gradually deposit on the inner walls of the arteries so that their bores are reduced and they lose their elasticity. A reduction of effective bore restricts the blood supply to tissues and organs and so makes it necessary for the heart and respiratory system to work harder to deliver the needed quantities of oxygen to the muscles. Loss of elasticity may lead to such weakening of an artery that it can stretch to form an aneurysm which may burst, or interfere with surrounding organs. The deposition of atheroma sometimes results in the formation of a clot (thrombus) which may be carried along in the bloodstream and cause a sudden constriction or even closure in an artery. If this happens in the coronary artery (which supplies blood to the heart) the coronary thrombosis reduces or cuts off the blood supply to part of the heart muscle and the victim suffers a heart attack, or myocardial infarction, which may well be fatal. This is the commonest cause both of death and of severe illness among middle aged men. The mechanism of cerebral thrombosis is similar. If a diseased blood vessel in the head ruptures, the result is a cerebral haemorrhage, which may cause permanent brain damage.

Clearly the first step towards reducing the prospect of heart attack is to discover the cause of the degenerative changes in the blood vessels. There are two main approaches: more intensive physiological research into the biological mechanism of these changes, and continuous search for a statistical correlation between the illnesses these changes cause and factors such as age, sex, heredity, diet, occupation, smoking, physical exercise, psychological stress and the effects of other illnesses. The number of possible factors is so large that the analysis of data is very difficult and is still inconclusive. The influence of heredity is firmly established: if both parents have coronary heart disease the risk of their son suffering a coronary thrombosis in his turn is increased nearly five fold. Sex is also an established variable: nearly twice as many men as women die because of a coronary thrombosis. It is reasonable to seek a link with diet because diet determines, at least to some extent, the nature and levels of fat in the blood and because excessive body mass demands extra work from the heart and lungs. Smoking, too, might be expected to increase the risk because of possible lung damage and because absorption of carbon monoxide from tobacco smoke into the blood reduces its capacity to absorb and transport oxygen. Regular exercise seems to reduce the risk, and this might be expected since it helps to keep the respiratory and circulatory organs working efficiently. But sudden and unusual exercise may be fatal in someone with unsuspected degenerative disease.

This discussion does not imply that the details of heart diseases should be taught in schools, but suggests that a shift of emphasis when respiration, circulation and nutrition are explained can illustrate that biology supports the commonsense view that, within the wide limits imposed on us all by our genes, the most effective way of reducing the prospect of heart attack consists in moderation in our life-style and in keeping fit.

Nearly all girls, and many boys, are taught at school that food contains carbohydrates, proteins, fats, vitamins and mineral elements, all essential to health. They learn that these substances are present in different proportions in different foods so that balanced meals are needed to ensure that adequate quantities of each are consumed. They also learn in simple terms the principles of the digestive process. These matters are discussed in a number of well-known text books, including publications from recent curriculum development teams—see references and suggestions for further reading.

In England and Wales plentiful supplies of a wide variety of foods are available so we are not dependent on one single food for an essential nutriment. Choice of food is determined by individual taste, family preference, and social custom. The range of choice is so wide that serious deficiency in a vital element is uncommon, but cases of undernutrition in children can occur as a result of ignorance and mismanagement. Similar reasons are the cause of the rarer malnutrition in adults. Alcoholics, for example, disregard the need for a balanced food intake.

The amount of nutriment available to the body to keep it in optimum health depends on the quantity and nature of the food. The protein and carbohydrate needed for growth and energy depend on how much the body requires at any one time. Demand is relatively high during growth, including pregnancy, and among those who do heavy manual work, while it is relatively low in middle age and among those who have sedentary jobs. A relatively high intake of protein and vitamins is necessary in old age when there may be a falling off in the efficiency of the body's metabolic processes.

The weight of an adult varies little from year to year or even from decade to decade if he remains healthy. But when people persist in eating and drinking in excess of their needs, the balance is laid down as fat and so they become obese. This may happen because ingrained eating habits continue when the energy need has fallen, or as a result of compulsive eating, a neurotic state of obsession with food. Obesity can occur in children simply because they are given too much to eat, but there are diseases that cause overweight.

Obesity is very much commoner in westernised countries than undernutrition and is more difficult to define than recognise, because a quantitative definition implies a correct weight for every individual in the world. The certain result of obesity, as has been mentioned earlier in connection with heart disease, is a demand for extra work from the heart and lungs to move the larger mass. Also, deposits of fat are laid down in muscle tissue, making the muscles less efficient. Obesity has the possible effect in some middle-aged people of hastening the onset of dieseases such as heart attacks and diabetes.

Weight can be lost only by reducing the food intake, especially of those foods with a high content of carbohydrate. Only the strong-willed succeed because the body is used to and enjoys its habitual intake of food and drink. Many schemes have been devised to make dieting as painless as possible by altering the proportions as well as the quantities of nutriments, sometimes in ways that greatly increase the cost, but energy-reduced foods still contain energy. Efforts are made to lose weight for health and for cosmetic reasons. Dieting which involves a radical change in the amount and type of food, designed to give a rapid reduction in weight, should never be undertaken without medical supervision.

Gross underweight is rare and is almost always a symptom or consequence of disease. Excessive slimming in girls and young women may lead to *anorexia nervosa*, a self-induced food aversion which may be a sign of difficulty in adjusting to the prospect of adult life. This may induce changes in the hormone control system which make it physically very difficult to reverse the process. Whatever the causes, *anorexia nervosa* is recognised as a grave illness.

These brief comments on nutrition point again to the distinction between science and health education. Despite all the teaching in schools and an abundance of accurate attractively presented information in magazines and newspapers, obesity is common. But health education is, among other things, about behaviour, which is often apparently irrational. Like the discussion of heart disease, the topic of obesity illustrates the difficulty of enabling boys and girls who do not study biology in depth to appreciate the interrelation between the systems (respiration, circulation and so on) and the problem of organising the very large number of biological facts into a body of useful knowledge; so much effort is needed to learn the facts that little capacity is left for learning to apply relevant facts to a given health hazard. But perhaps a natural interest in human health and disease may encourage learning.

Various curriculum development programmes have suggested ways in which biological knowledge can be organised. The Biological Sciences Curriculum Study material from the United States has indicated that biological concepts can be associated with many levels of organisation—molecule; cell; tissue organism; ecosystem. There are many biological ideas at each of these levels. It is an interesting exercise to see how they can be extended into health topics, bearing in mind that health education is concerned with prevention and understanding rather than with a morbid preoccupation with disease—that is, with health rather than with sickness. The associated table provides an example of what can result from such an exercise. Readers may be interested to complete the table by filling in the empty column—knowledge apart from biology needed in health topics.

Enough has been written to suggest that the relationship between biology and health education can also be looked at as part of the controversy between a subject approach and integrated studies in schools. The observed fact that biological knowledge alone does not necessarily improve health behaviour suggests that one method of using biological and other knowledge for health education might be to group topics into situational exercises. For example, what action might be expected of someone telephoning a doctor; preparing food for a family; trying to regulate the size of the family; someone who suspects an abnormal pregnancy; who wishes to lose weight; who wishes to stop smoking;

Level of organisation	biological concepts	some examples of health topics	knowledge apart from biology needed in health topics
Molecule	essential mineral salts vitamins amino acids	varied diet	
Cell	poisonous substances eg mercury carcinogens	occupational hazards	
	antigen—antibody	immunisation	
	genes	genetic conselling	
	cell differentiation	growth and control of growth wound healing cancer	
Tissue	skeleton	dental health & foot health and posture fractures and X-ray	
	circulatory system	effects of exercise first aid cardiovascular malfunctions eg coronary disease; thrombosis; varicose veins bloodgroups; Rh factor *Haemophilia*	
	muscle/nerve	physical co-ordination, PE and effects of exercise effects of drugs and alcohol nervous and muscular disease eg tetanus, poliomyelitis	
	sense organs	defects of eyesight and hearing	
	respiratory system	bronchitis; effects of smoking and pollution occupational hazards resuscitation	
	digestive system	diet; digestive rhythms indigestion	
	hormones	effects of adrenalin control of diabetes the contraceptive pill	
Organism	growth and development	stages of foetal and child growth	
	variation	individual variation eg onset of puberty	
	behaviour	aggression courtship child care and stress	

Level of organisation	biological concepts	some examples of health topics	knowledge apart from biology needed in health topics
Ecosystems	cycles of activity	circadian rhythms sleep menstrual cycle and contraception	
	food-chains	concentration of DDT in man	
	agricultural productivity	vegetable textured protein and the 'green revolution'	
	host/parasite	infectious diseases control of malaria	
	energy relationships	world food resources, famine and obesity	

who has to withstand a period of high pressure at work? A look at such situations will lead to team work and interdisciplinary study in which the biologist has an important role. Developments of this kind are to be seen in some secondary schools, where health education is regarded not as an isolated subject but as an emerging structure of facts and ideas from many subjects related to health.

A brief mention has been made of growth. The importance to teachers and parents of physical growth, especially the variations in the time and the speed of the changes that occur between infancy and manhood, will be emphasised at several points in this pamphlet. Thanks to the work of J M Tanner and others (see references) the stages of human physical growth have been thoroughly observed and are now well understood, while the biological mechanism is gradually being unravelled. Growth is a matter of cell division (replication), of cell differentiation, and of cell replacement. Most important, it is a matter of control, a very complicated programme which involves automatic triggering of a series of changes and stopping them at the proper times. If this control breaks down, undifferentiated tissue develops into a 'growth', which may be benign, or malignant (as in cancer). Many of these ideas are at least in outline appropriate, and reassuring, for boys and girls as well as for their teachers and parents. Such a biological basis can provide the essential scientific discipline in the increasing range of courses offered in secondary schools on child development or education for parenthood.

References

Molecules to man Biological Sciences Curriculum Study, Edward Arnold, 1963.

Further reading

'The Endocrine Glands: an introductory sketch.' Ch. 18 in *The thinking machine*, J Brierley, Heinemann, 1973.

'Hormones and Genes' in *The scientific American*, E H Davidson, Scientific American, June, 1965.

'Diseases of Civilisation—Blood Vessels' Ch. 23 in *Man against disease*, A G Clegg and P C Clegg, Heinemann, 1973.

Education and physical growth, J M Tanner, ULP, 1961.

Growth at adolescence (2nd Edition), J M Tanner, Blackwell, 1969.

'Hormone, Genetic and Environmental Factors Controlling Growth', Ch. 21 in *Human biology*, G A Harrison, J S Weiner, J M Tanner and N A Barnicott, OUP, 1964.

'The Regulation of Living Processes' Ch. 8 in **Molecules and cells*, D A Coult, Longmans, 1966.

*Heart drugs—the chemical control of heart function, ICI, ICI Educational Publications, 1974.

Examples of biological problems related to health education, in *Biology teachers' handbook*, J J Schwab (Ed.), Wiley (New York), 1963.

Biology of Man (Secondary Science III), Nuffield Foundation, Longmans, 1971.

'Digestion and Absorption', Ch. 5 in *Maintenance of the organism* (Biological, Science), Nuffield Foundation, Penguin 1971.

'Food and Digestion', in *The maintenance of life* (Biology III), Nuffield Foundation, Longmans, 1966.

Food and the principles of nutrition (12th edition), Sir R Hutchinson and Dean Moncrieff, Edward Arnold, 1969.

*'Obesity' in the *British medical journal* vol. I pp 560–563, J Anderson, 1972.

Obesity: medical and scientific aspects, I M Baird and A N Howard (Eds.), E and S Livingstone, 1969.

Human nutrition (2nd Edition), V H Mottram, Edward Arnold, 1972.

4

HEALTH EDUCATION IN SCHOOLS

Health education is neither recognised, nor recognisable, in the school curriculum in the sense that mathematics is recognised and recognisable. But health education is unavoidable, even if its presence is denied. The infant teacher who instructs her charges in the appropriate times to wash their hands; the primary teacher who introduces boys and girls to the ways in which animals and human beings organise themselves to care for their young; teachers in secondary schools who discuss with their pupils Mozart's operas, or the properties of sulphur dioxide, or the conservation of resources or the elements of probability are all involved, whether they realise it or not. Their influence may be greater than they suppose. If so ancient an educational aim as the development of a healthy mind in a healthy body is accepted, the contributions of teachers of all expressive and creative arts, and of gymnastics, games and sports are self-evident. Such teachers also help to maintain a healthy mind in a healthy body throughout life when they arouse interests which grow into absorbing leisure activities, which may include physical skills and exercise as well as the creativity of the craftsman. So in a fragmented way health education happens to boys and girls in all schools without anyone necessarily being aware of its totality. Nowadays, however, a growing number of schools adopt a more positive approach.

Assessment is very difficult, and inspection of some aspects of health education may illustrate one of the basic tenets of quantum physics: that observation of a physical system disturbs it. There is often no recognisable way in which success may be measured: sometimes there is no consensus of what constitutes success. On the other hand, failure in some aspects of health education is all too readily apparent and all too quickly pointed out. No one can measure the value of the right words from teacher to pupil at the right time: words which carry conviction in proportion to the pupil's assessment of the integrity and understanding of the teacher. The qualities in teachers which inspire this confidence sometimes defy analysis. There are occasions when to find the right reassuring or explanatory words may demand the skills of the counsellor or even those of the psychotherapist.

Probably the main stimulus for recent developments in health education in schools, especially secondary schools, is the wish, seen by many adults as a duty, to protect boys and girls from hazards to their health created by their own behaviour. Individuals and groups organised to propagate various attitudes to these hazards have sometimes forgotten, to quote the Crowther report (see Chapter 14), that education can only function within the broad directives of right and wrong which society gives.

Another stimulus is the growing realisation that health education, at one time thought of as no more than a matter of hygiene—as a simple matter of sanitation, clean water, fresh air, adequate diet and exercise—is now seen to be not so simple but to raise difficult questions of individual and social behaviour, and to depend on knowledge belonging to several disciplines. For example, is water which has a concentration of one part per million of fluoride ions pure? What are acceptable levels of carbon monoxide, sulphur dioxide, or tetra ethyl lead in the air and how can they be monitored and controlled? What is an adequate diet for an English factory worker or a Japanese company director; and why? Is the fostering of the qualities of courage, fitness, balance, and persistence revealed by a boy who has the makings of a good scrum half to be discouraged because all boys do not possess them? These are important questions and each demands a rational answer.

In the infant or first school, as in the primary school and at least the earlier years of the middle school, there is no dichotomy between pastoral care and teaching. On the contrary the physical, emotional, social and intellectual development of each child is seen as a whole, a viewpoint which is highly favourable for the beginnings of health education. The health education of young children consists to a large extent in the acceptance of values by example and the learning of behaviour, including elements of training, from good practice. The influence, depending on the attitudes of every teacher as well as the caretaker, members of the school meals staff and playground supervisors, is inescapable. Teaching may for convenience be grouped under many headings, for example, Myself, Other People, and the Environment; but there is no suggestion that any such broad groups should be separated from one another or isolated from the rest of the curriculum. But changes of emphasis, some as a reaction to the crisis topics which disturb the secondary school, are to be seen.

The experimental introduction a few years ago of the BBC Merry Go Round programmes on human birth and reproduction has influenced health education in many primary schools. Among their effects has been a significant increase in co-operation and understanding between many teachers and parents. It is noticeable that in schools where these programmes have been used for some years they are nowadays shown to younger and younger children. Interest in science in the primary school —especially revealed by such books as *Ourselves* by the Schools Council Project Science 5–13 (see references)—have encouraged teachers to introduce children to simple ideas of growth, variation, and how their bodies work. Changes in religious teaching have perhaps made clearer to children the interdependence of us all, the variety both of family and social customs, and of ethical beliefs which impinge on health. The following two extracts from reports written by one of HM Inspectors a few years ago describe experiments by teachers of older primary children. Whether similar developments are appropriate in the context of their own work is solely for the individual teacher to decide.

'The headmaster decided to combine two classes (third and fourth year juniors) to work for three to four hours a week for a term on a health project. The course began with a descriptive treatment of the skeletal system, muscles and organs of the body followed by grouping of children to study a particular part and report to the main group. Parents were soon heavily involved and were, according to the headmaster, often badgered by their children for information. Books began to arrive in the school, the local butcher provided various spare parts for examination and a nearby university department loaned appropriate models.

After this "medical" foundation had been laid the boys and girls watched the BBC Merry Go Round sex education programmes. The headmaster attributes the sensible way in which these were received in part to the earlier stages of the project, and reported that the parents, quick to provide "feed back", were very pleased that their children had been so well informed and were delighted at the level and tone of the discussions and questions which had arisen at home following the programmes.

For the duration of the project each week one or two visitors to the school, (including a public health officer, a nurse, a school medical officer, a local general practitioner, the health education officer, a Red Cross training officer and the matron of a maternity hospital) spoke to the children and stood up to their searching questions.

The project ended with a display for parents of the children's work, including a film made in school. At the end of the experiment the teachers agreed that they had learned that primary children have a marked interest in human biology; that they are all capable of sustaining their interest in such a project; that they like adult visitors to address them as adults; that they respond with questions at a level which surprises and delights both speakers and teachers; and that a health project is an effective setting for the sex education programme.'

And, at another school:

'Interest in health education arose as a response to the dangers of smoking even among children under 11. But the headmaster decided, in consultation with parents, to explore the uses of the ITV programme "Living and Growing". He also decided not to treat this in isolation, but to regard simple study of the human life cycle as the culmination of a programme of work on the family and the community. There has evolved, for the boys and girls in their fourth year, a two-term course called "The Family—a Social and Biological Study", taught by an experienced woman member of the staff and the headmaster. Emphasis is placed on the notions of the roles, responsibilities and needs of various members of the family, and then, in a community such as a school, the need for security, consideration for others, and for some rules of conduct. The human family is contrasted with the methods adopted by various animals in caring for their young, and a wide range of legends, stories and modern writing is woven into the scheme. Consideration is then given to the way in which human beings function, the senses, the digestive system (with a glance at the beginnings of nutrition) structure (with a look at a dissected rat—not dissected in front of the boys and girls), and breathing, including a simple study of the atmosphere and references to air pollution and to smoking. The work is concluded by reference to the human life cycle, including introductory discussion of inherited characteristics such as tongue curling and eye colour.'

Caution is needed not to simplify the elements of human biology so drastically that they become absurd. It is not unknown for children to be given the outlines of the circulation of the blood with no hint of the purpose of so elaborate an arrangement, or for the digestive system to be presented in such a way that food and drink appear to be put in at one end and emitted unchanged at the other.

In the past decade about 50 local education authorities have published the findings of working parties set up to advise teachers in their schools on health education. These working parties have invariably included teachers and medical officers with advisory and administrative officials, and usually others such as health visitors, health education officers, social workers and police officers. They have changed from being concerned exclusively with one aspect, such as sex education in secondary schools, to wider considerations of health education. Their conclusions have often been presented as ingredients in broad programmes of social education, moral education and pastoral care for schools of all kinds, with emphasis on the needs of adolescent boys and girls. They have never proposed extraordinary and isolated attention to topics of current concern, but have attempted to weave these into broad patterns of health education. Some have analysed the contributions of the subjects of the secondary curriculum. Many have listed topics judged appropriate for various age groups and have pointed to the departments in the school responsible for dealing with them.

Health education is implemented in secondary schools in a variety of ways which are shown in several forms of organisation which have emerged in the past few years. These include the following:

A. Health education is seen solely as a responsibility for subject teachers to discharge as they see fit, with possibly the addition of lectures by visitors, and talks, perhaps by a doctor or marriage guidance counsellor, to the girls.

B. A senior teacher, or group of senior teachers which may include the counsellor, is responsible for identifying, encouraging and co-ordinating aspects of health education in the traditional subject areas. Where this is done there may also be courses, compulsory or optional, on personal relationships and related topics, partly because the subject contributions, although regarded as vital, are seen not to be comprehensive.

C. Health education is a timetabled subject—not necessarily for all years—in the hands of a specialist teacher.
D. Health education is the responsibility of the counsellor or, if there is no counsellor, of year tutors.

Which of these patterns is established (and two or more may exist concurrently) clearly depends on the aims and the circumstances of the school. There is no question of any one of them being universally right while all others are wrong. There is a little evidence (some of the experiments are very recent), on which no more than a few cautious comments can safely rest.

A. has little to commend it, but it is still adopted, perhaps most often in selective schools.

B., as has been stated earlier, is the commonest recent development. It makes great demands on the knowledge, on the tact, and on the effective diplomacy of senior teachers who act as co-ordinators. Perhaps its greatest merit is that it encourages teachers to look at their subjects from another point of view. But it is difficult, as has been pointed out in Chapter 3, to reorient biology (and, no doubt, other subjects) towards health education, and attempts to do so may be as superficial as efforts to make physics seem useful by mentioning to every generation of boys and girls Archimedes' reaction to his famous observation. Advocates of B. fairly claim that duplication may be avoided. This needs a little care as there are advantages in presenting the same topic to pupils at different points in their school career because they vary in the pace at which they approach maturity, and there is gain when topics in health education are studied from different perspectives. Teachers also know that the best lessons sometimes arise from the skilful and spontaneous exploitation of apparent irrelevance.

C., which is adopted by very few schools partly because so few teachers have appropriate specialist qualifications, has the attractiveness of tidiness. But it still further fragments the curriculum, disregards contributions from other teachers, and may even encourage the invention of yet more subjects for public examination, while the unfortunate teacher responsible for perhaps 30 classes has a poor prospect of getting to know his pupils very well.

D. gives opportunity for boys and girls to discuss health education in an informal way with a counsellor or teacher who can get to know them well. This may help counsellors and teachers to detect early signs of disturbance. It may, however, emphasise the protective aspect of health education at the expense of its academic content, and suggest to boys and girls a rigid distinction between the teaching and pastoral functions of teachers. Of course health education cannot be divorced from pastoral care; nor can mathematics or French.

Whatever arrangements are adopted, important conditions to be satisfied are that health education is limited neither to one or two years nor to only some of the boys and girls, and that the knowledge and ideas the pupils bring from their previous schools are not ignored.

Courses called 'Education in Personal Relationships', or 'Social Education', or 'Education for Parenthood', or even 'Education for Life' are appearing in many secondary schools and include aspects of health education, especially sex. Such titles may prompt the cynical question: what is the function of the rest of the work of the school if not for these very purposes? But these developments are a reaction of many experienced teachers, stimulated no doubt by some LEA working parties, to a growing belief that something more than haphazard pastoral care is needed and that scholarship—which includes the sum of human self-knowledge, human experience and human skills—is not always seen by boys and girls to provide the answers to problems which may beset them, now or in the future. The danger of superficiality is obvious. Education for parenthood, for example, is concerned with the total development of the personality, not merely the skills of infant care, and an important practical need of young parents is to know when, where and from whom to seek advice as they try to get on with the job. Being a good parent— a more difficult notion to define than to recognise—implies an ability to cope with life and the sensitivity to realise that children educate and influence their parents. The test of all these courses is threefold. First, the extent to which, to return to a quotation in Chapter I, they succeed in being more than collections of barren facts which do not germinate and so produce nothing in a boy or girl's mind. Secondly, the extent to which they include more than casual discussions of complex ideas. Thirdly, the extent to which they capture the attention of boys and girls, and develop their self knowledge, self confidence, and awareness of others. Teachers who are not involved in such courses must never be allowed to believe that they have no pastoral role.

The appointment of school counsellors in secondary schools began in the early 1960's. Such appointments are nowadays increasingly common but far from universal. Almost invariably the school counsellor is a qualified teacher with training in counselling and in other aspects of the practice of guidance in education. Sometimes he (or she) is an experienced teacher who has become involved in health education and who feels the need for more knowledge and skill in responding to difficulties which boys and girls sometimes reveal; so he may qualify as a counsellor and return to his school. It is an advantage to a school counsellor to be known and respected by his colleagues in the common room as a skilful and successful teacher.

The training of counsellors sometimes includes a substantial study of health education. If they are then appointed to schools as teacher-counsellors they may well be responsible for devising programmes in personal relationships, or sex education, or vocational development which do not, as we have earlier seen, slot easily into a traditional curriculum framework. Thus while a counsellor always has an important indirect role to play in health education it is sometimes an important direct role.

The majority of boys and girls are sufficiently resilient and fortunate in their homes and in their friends to survive, and often enjoy, growing up. They do so successfully with the help, encouragement and understanding of teachers who are not seen by them as mere providers of information. But some children meet problems which need more attention than can be given during a brief talk between teacher and pupil. Break up of the home is an example. There may also be acute anxiety over transitory difficulties which some adults, who have forgotten what it is like to be 15, see as trivial. The counsellor is enabled by his training and experience to listen and eventually (in most cases) to ensure that the child grows through the problem in the knowledge and confidence that it has no permanent significance. There may be more serious difficulties such as injury, sometimes criminal, inflicted on children, or a breach of the law by the child. In such cases the counsellor has not only to counsel but to decide whom to consult.

In many secondary schools a few boys and girls have great difficulty in accepting anything which the school offers because they cannot relate to adults or to the majority of their contemporaries. They are seriously disturbed. The counsellor's function is to recognise their need, arrange for diagnosis and treatment by those qualified to undertake it, and eventually to play a major part in the extremely difficult task of rehabilitating them in the school.

Boys and girls have many ways of showing that they need help, ranging from dramatic and unmistakable outbursts of temper or of violence to withdrawal or a decline in the standards of their work. The counsellor is trained to recognise these signals and to help his colleagues to do so. He is also concerned to minimise the chances of abrasive contacts or misunderstandings which may aggravate distress. Ways in which schools can seek to reduce the risks of excessive stress and transient mental ill-health are discussed in Chapter 11 in relation to the misuse of drugs. The counsellor has a contribution to make in these efforts.

Counselling is a process by which boys and girls are helped to become more aware of the possibilities available to them and is particularly concerned with helping them to see constructive possibilities when a daunting problem is standing in the way. The counsellor cannot escape the ethical implications of his work. His business is with individuals, not with reforming society, so his ethical stance is the agreed stance of the school. He works by helping his colleagues to become more competent in reading and interpreting behaviour; by helping those who come to him, whether because their work and behaviour is causing concern to themselves or to others, or because they are aware of a need to discuss and explore their personal problems in private. He is an important link between the school and its doctor, its educational psychologist, its child psychiatrist, the parents and the responsible social workers. He needs above all emotional detachment and the humility to recognise when he does not know.

Curriculum Paper No 14, *Health education in schools*, published by the Scottish Education Department in 1974, included in its advice about sex education a few paragraphs on the presentation of sexual knowledge to handicapped pupils. In particular this paper drew attention to the problems of children suffering from spina bifida, with the advice that they should not be excluded from the normal programmes of sex education given to their class mates. It also pointed out that great care must be taken to ensure that mentally handicapped girls are prepared for menstruation, and mentioned special difficulty in sex education for the blind. The Scottish working party concluded that the problems of handicapped pupils require particular and separate consideration and they recommended that an enquiry be instituted.

Children receiving special education and those with a degree of physical or mental handicap being educated in ordinary schools fall into three broad groups with respect to their needs for health education: those with sensory and physical disabilities; those with learning difficulties which may include a degree of mental subnormality; and those with difficulties in making relationships and in their social adjustment.

For the first group continuous medical supervision coupled with a variety of therapies will ensure the supervision of their health and some instruction in personal health and hygiene. But health education as such may not be a marked feature of their curriculum. For many the content may be similar to that for other children but the way it is taught to them may need to be modified.

The second group requires careful selection of what is taught and modification of the methods of presentation. So far as is known very little work has been done on schemes of health education appropriate for severely subnormal pupils.

The third group of maladjusted and delinquent children has particular needs. Often, the education of children in this group includes an element involving consideration of human relationships. This is an aspect of health education of growing importance because advances in medical knowledge will increasingly enable handicapped children not only to survive but to take a constructive place in society. A great deal has still to be learned.

Health education is a part of the work of teachers which they share with parents to a greater degree than perhaps is apparent in other aspects of their job. Throughout health education there is an immediately protective element, with a growing scholarly element which is essential in order that health studies may be seen as a necessary part of a liberal education and so may contribute to helping boys and girls to become men and women whose health is founded on an understanding of themselves and a knowledge of the services provided by the community.

The beginnings of understanding spring from the home, supplemented and gradually deepened in the school. This joint responsibility, especially to young children, is becoming recognised as fundamental to health education, and suggests that probably the single most effective field for the deployment of medical skills in health education is in the education of parents of very young children. Such education is more likely to succeed if young parents have been so educated at school and at home that they are receptive to the continuing need for health education, and capable of unearthing relevant information for themselves as well as seeking, and understanding, medical advice.

Teachers need not only knowledge of what they teach as health education but knowledge which enables them to protect children by drawing the attention of doctors to incipient physical and emotional problems which they are able to spot. They need to know what they must know to understand growing children, and to know what they must teach to help the children eventually to understand themselves.

Uncritical enthusiasm for health education may sometimes ignore second order effects (see Chapter 7). For example, in discussion of the prevention of smoking among young people, parents and older brothers are sometimes said to be the key to young children's attitudes to smoking, while the adolescent peer group is also said to be a powerful influence. It follows that smoking might be substantially reduced in the next generation by isolating some children from their families and by encouraging solitary behaviour in adolescents. The practical absurdity of this conclusion points to the necessity for a sense of proportion in health education and to the danger in considering one problem in isolation. The reader may think of other instances where lack of informed common sense, which often in practice means failure to predict second order effects, may tempt the health educator to cross the line which separates the enthusiast from the crank.

Further reading

Child development—physical and psychological development through adolescence (5th Edition), M E Breckenridge and E L Vincent, Saunders, 1965.

'Human Growth and Constitution' Pt. IV in *Human biology*, G A Harrison, J S Weiner, J M Tanner and N A Barnicott, OUP, 1964.

Growth and development of children (5th Edition), E H Watson and G H Lourey, Year Book Medical Publishers, 1967.

Education and physical growth, J M Tanner, ULP, 1961.

Growth at adolescence (2nd Edition), J M Tanner, Blackwell, 1969.

Ourselves, stages 1 and 2 (Science 5–13), Schools Council, Macdonald Educational, 1973.

'Effect of Televised Sex Education at the Primary School Level', Ch. 18 in *Sex education: rationale and reaction*, R S Rogers (Ed.), CUP, 1974.

'Guidance as a Concept in Educational Theory', (Ch. 5) 'Teaching in its Personal Context', (Ch. 7) in *Objectives and perspectives in education*, B Morris, Routledge and Kegan Paul, 1972.

'Social, Emotional, and Personality Development', Ch. 6 in *Readings in the foundation of education*, W F Connell, R L Debus and W R Niblett, Routledge and Kegan Paul, 1967.

Education and the concept of mental health, J Wilson, Routledge and Kegan Paul, 1969.

'Development and Mental Health', Ch. 2 in *Mental health and the education process*, H F Clarizio (Ed.), Rand McNally, 1969.

'Health Education in Schools', (Ch. 9) 'Health Education Through Other Subjects', (Ch. 10) in *A textbook of health education*, Dr A J Dalzell-Ward, Tavistock Publications, 1974.

The faith of the counsellors, P Halmos, Constable, 1965.

School counselling in practice, A Jones, Ward Lock, 1970.

Counselling, Lady Venables, NMGC, 1971.

Guidance and counselling in schools: a response to change, P M Hughes, Pergamon, 1971.

Counselling in schools, K D Bradshaw, HMA and NACE, 1973.

School counselling (Working party report), NAMH, 1970.

5

COMMUNICABLE DISEASES

The effects of improved sanitation, better nutrition, less overcrowding, and the developments of immunisation and of antibiotics in reducing, and in some instances virtually stopping, deaths in industrialised countries from infectious and contagious diseases were mentioned in Chapter 1. In England and Wales today a great deal of illness is still caused by viral infections, as is shown in Table V. In tropical and sub-tropical regions, malaria, sleeping sickness, bilharzia and other diseases remain the main causes of death or debility while outbreaks of cholera, rabies, typhus and plague are not unknown, even in more temperate parts of the world.

Some understanding of the causes, transmission, spread, control, cure and the prospects of the eventual elimination of communicable diseases is important to everyone. Control is very much a matter of individual as well as collective responsibility. Translation from science to sensible action is often simple and almost obvious in this part of health education. Science teaching should enable boys and girls to understand, for example, why portions of uncooked chicken stored close to a pork pie in a refrigerator can cause food poisoning when the pie is eaten. They should also realise from their biology lessons that the virtual elimination of a childhood disease such as diphtheria does not imply that the proper immunisation is no longer necessary; that diseases and their distribution patterns change so that vigilance is still needed; that the great advances in chemotherapy do not lessen the importance of personal and public hygiene; and that resistance to many illnesses which may not be fatal but which are certainly a nuisance is still largely a matter of keeping the body well maintained by sensible diet, adequate sleep and exercise.

For many years boys and girls have been taught simple ideas about germs and the spread of disease. They often learn about van Leeuwenhoek and his 'little animals'; how Pasteur showed that some microorganisms are responsible for fermentation and how he and Koch proved that others cause anthrax; the stories of Edward Jenner and of Sir Alexander Fleming. Very few boys and girls leave school without having seen at least a picture of Pasteur's celebrated swan-neck flasks, although some may be a little vague about the reasons for their shape. Recently, encouraged by the curriculum developments of the sixties, boys and girls have been introduced to elementary experiments with microbes and it is now becoming exceptional to find a secondary school where, at some stage, the pupils do not cultivate bacteria and moulds on nutritive jellies.

The living organisms which cause communicable diseases include, in order of size, viruses, bacteria, fungi (moulds and yeasts), protozoa, worms and other minute animals which may prey on man, his crops or his livestock. These various organisms invade the human body and the bodies of other animals and co-exist with their hosts, on whom and in whom they sometimes live permanently. Some, such as the bacteria which live in man's intestines and produce some of the B vitamins and vitamin K, may be essential for the well-being of their host. Some are harmless. Others may cause vague and slowly deteriorating ill health for many years. A few may cause death within a matter of hours. Total destruction of all bacteria is impossible, and if it could be achieved would soon result in the death of all living things.

In England and Wales worms are a very minor hazard because of the very high standards of hygiene insisted on in the supply of meat, especially pork, for human consumption. However thread worms (*Enterobius vermicularis*) are common and many children are infested at times. They can cause intense anal irritation, especially at night, and so disturb sleep.

The protozoa include many free-living animals such as *Amoeba proteus*, well known to most boys and girls. One form, *Entamoeba histolytica*, may live in the large intestine and cause amoebic dysentery, a very rare disease in this country. Others cause several forms of sleeping sickness, endemic in tropical Africa. Members of the *Plasmodium* species are responsible for malaria. These organisms have complicated life cycles involving a secondary host, often a blood-sucking insect, which distributes the parasites to new primary hosts. They are of great importance in tropical medicine but of little significance in temperate areas. They are usually attacked by destroying the secondary hosts.

The fungi are plant-like though they lack the green pigment chlorophyll and are thus unable to manufacture their own food using sunlight as the source of energy. Instead, they use complex substances as food so that many of them are important in the processes of natural decay and in the deterioration of stored foods. A few live on or in man and may cause illness. They produce large numbers of spores which are dispersed by air currents and become a normal constituent of dust. Ringworm and athlete's foot are fungal infections of the skin; thrush results from a yeast-like fungal infection of mucous surfaces in the mouth and in the vagina.

Bacteria are larger than viruses and were discovered earlier, because viruses are too small to be seen with an optical microscope. Bacteria have simple structures and as only their shape is clearly discernible with a microscope this is the characteristic by which they are named and classified. For example, the cocci are spherical or ellipsoidal with a diameter of the order of one micrometre. The staphylococci appear in bunches; the streptococci arrange themselves in chains like a necklace of beads; the diplococci appear in pairs. The bacilli are rodlike; the vibrios are comma shaped; and the spirillae are long and corkscrew shaped.

The number and variety of bacteria are enormous. They colonise air, water and soil, as well as the outsides and the insides of our bodies and the bodies of other living things. Many of them are essential since they directly break down the bodies of dead animals and plants and help in the disposal of sewage. They are used in cheesemaking, in fermentation and brewing, in composting, and in attacking disease organisms using chemical substances (antigens) produced by some of them. It is quite misleading to leave boys and girls with the impression that bacteria are invariably the enemy of man: on the contrary we cannot survive without them, and it is therefore vital that they should not be indiscriminately destroyed. However, a few are pathogenic (or in some circumstances may become so) when they may cause diseases such as scarlet fever, diphtheria, tuberculosis, food poisoning, tetanus, plague, cholera, gonorrhoea, leprosy, and boils. Such bacteria excrete harmful toxins as products of their living processes. Some toxins are released continuously, others only when the bacteria have died. Some toxins, unlike bacteria, are resistant to high temperatures and may survive in re-heated food causing food poisoning.

Bacteria reproduce by dividing into two, as frequently as every 20 minutes in the most favourable conditions of warmth and food supply, and an immense population can build up in a few hours. Like other living organisms they show occasional spontaneous changes from generation to generation, called mutations, which are relatively very frequent compared with mutations in man because of the very much greater rate of reproduction. Some mutants may show increased vigour or increased resistance to different environments so that the virulence of a disease may change, and strains which are resistant to a previously effective antibiotic may appear.

Viruses are extremely small, with diameters in the range 30–300 nanometres, and can be seen only by using an electron microscope. Many are small enough to pass through bacteria-proof filters. Like bacteria they exist in many varieties, multiply very rapidly in favourable conditions, and may mutate very frequently. Unlike bacteria they are able to reproduce only in living cells and must colonise the cells of their host in order to multiply sufficiently to cause disease. They are therefore generally more difficult than bacteria to attack when in the body because they are more intimately linked with it. They are also more difficult to investigate experimentally because they have to be cultured in the laboratory within the cells of incubated living eggs. They cause, among other diseases, measles, mumps, chicken pox, rubella (German measles), whooping cough, influenza, the common cold, poliomyelitis and warts—some of which (for example, measles, rubella in the foetus, and poliomyelitis) may leave permanent damage because of the destruction of cells by the invading viruses. There is also growing evidence that certain viruses induce cancers in animals under experimental conditions.

Viruses and bacteria which cause infections can be transmitted from the source of infection to their next victims by the breath, by sputum, milk, blood, skin, urine or faeces, and can invade directly, indirectly, or via an intermediate host. The most frequent mode of transmission is by direct contact with an infected person, the organisms gaining entry by being swallowed, inhaled or absorbed through a breach in the skin or mucous membrane. Infection is often spread by 'droplet infection' from the breath of a person suffering from a disease of the nose, throat or lungs. Whenever he breathes or talks, or still more when he coughs or sneezes, he propels into the air, for a distance of several feet, minute droplets of moisture which are heavily laden with germs. These organisms may then be inhaled, or settle on food or contaminate household or school articles being used by others. Food is particularly liable to become contaminated while it is being prepared by those who have an infection. An infected person may not have symptoms of the disease, or the symptoms may be so mild that he is unaware that he has been infected. Such a carrier may unknowingly harbour an infection for a long time and pass on virulent germs to others. Animals are frequently sources of infectious diseases either directly or indirectly from their products such as milk. A wide variety of animals excrete organisms which produce diseases in man such as food poisoning. Foodstuffs consumed by man which are contaminated by animals or insects may cause diseases. Rats are so notorious as contaminators of food that it is mandatory for every local authority to employ a rat catcher.

Hygiene is essentially a matter of limiting the distribution of micro-organisms which cause disease. Micro-organisms vary greatly in their ability to survive transmission. At one extreme the gonococcus responsible for gonorrhoea is a parasite which cannot survive except in contact with a human body so it can only be transmitted by sexual contacts. At the other extreme the bacteria which cause tetanus surround themselves with thick walls and thus become spores which are dispersed by air currents and resist destruction by heat or water loss, so they may survive in the soil for many years. When such spores enter the body through a wound the bacteria return to an environment in which they can multiply. Different methods of transmission explain why the grosser bacterial infections such as cholera and plague are virtually eliminated by efficient sanitation whereas colds, influenza and similar viral nuisances are still widely dispersed because we cough and sneeze. Another factor in the transmission of disease is the number of organisms needed to establish themselves in the host to cause disease—relatively very small for typhoid, very large for paratyphoid fever.

Whether or not a given host succumbs to a given disease depends on

several factors, such as the number of invading organisms; their virulence (which may change as they mutate); on the situation of the invading organisms (which may for example be harmless on the skin but
dangerous if introduced into normally sterile areas of the body by injury
or by surgery, which is why sterile conditions are essential in the operating
theatre); on the ability of the germs to spread through the host; and on
his power of resistance. Resistance varies from person to person, and
depends on whether the disease has been suffered before. Natural
resistance, or immunity, is enhanced by adequate rest and sleep, fresh
air and exercise, and by a balanced and varied diet: it is lowered by
fatigue, exposure to cold, and by intermittent illness, so that in a sense
some illness is cumulative and a bad habit.

The interval between the invasion of the organisms and the onset of
symptoms is called the incubation period of the disease. This is the period
when the germs are multiplying and producing effects in their victim.
During this time the person is often very infectious to others and it is
therefore important with some dangerous diseases (such as smallpox)
that the victim's contacts with others are noted if he is aware that he has,
or may have, the disease. The length of the incubation period varies
from disease to disease, and is obviously one of the factors which determines the rate of growth of an epidemic. The courses which diseases
may take also differ widely, from the spectacular sequence of events in
bubonic plague (which rapidly leads to death) to the slow, very gradual
and inexorably progressive disfigurement of untreated leprosy.

The spread of an infection is limited by identifying, isolating and
curing the source (ie detection and cure); by blocking the route of transmission (ie hygiene); by increasing the immunity of potential contacts
(ie immunisation and 'healthy' living); and by limiting over-crowding.
Identification of the disease and its source are matters for the physician
in association with the bacteriologist and the public health authorities.
It may be necessary to isolate the patient. Treatment is obviously aimed
at curing the patient as quickly as possible, in his interests and in the
interests of others. As was mentioned in Chapter 1, the prospects of
success are nowadays enhanced enormously by a wide and increasing
range of antibiotics, substances which cure by destroying germs inside
the body. Earlier methods of cure consisted essentially in encouraging
the body to mobilise its own defences.

Disinfection (the destruction of pathogenic micro-organisms outside
the body) varies, too, with the severity and type of infection. In the
common infections of childhood simple washing of clothes may be all
that is needed, while in more serious illnesses careful disinfection of all
clothing, bed linen and articles contaminated by the patient's excretions
is essential to prevent transmission of the micro-organisms. Contacts
of persons suffering from the more severe infectious diseases may have
to be quarantined: usually such contacts are members of the family but

with the more dangerous diseases the circle of possible contacts investigated may be enlarged. Food handlers either suffering from or in contact with a communicable disease may be forbidden to work until they are shown to be free from infection.

In the past it was customary to exclude pupils suffering from the common infectious diseases from school for long periods. This caused considerable loss of valuable educational time with little noticeable limitation of the spread of infection because in most of the diseases of childhood the period of greatest infectivity is in the last few days of the incubation period and shortly after the appearance of clinical signs. Over the years there has been a gradual relaxation in the regulations excluding contacts from school (see references). Children are particularly vulnerable to epidemics which are liable to spread quickly among large numbers of people who meet in one place, as at school. Efficient ventilation, good natural lighting, and high standards of hygiene help to limit the transmission of diseases to which children are prone. Good personal hygiene from an early age will help. The proper use of (preferably disposable) handkerchiefs will reduce droplet infection. Handwashing, especially after using the lavatory, will lessen the incidence of intestinal infections. Scrupulous cleanliness is mandatory for staff and for pupils dealing with the preparation and the service of school meals.

The third and perhaps the most important way of controlling an infectious disease is to increase the immunity of potential victims. Any foreign protein (including bacteria and viruses which do not occur naturally in the body) acts as an antigen, causing cells in the bone marrow, the spleen, the liver, the lungs, the lymph glands or the small bowel to generate another protein called an antibody which circulates in the bloodstream. Each antigen triggers the formation of its own specific antibody. Each type of bacterium or virus contains several proteins; infection creates a set of several antibodies in a combination specific to the invading micro-organism. When antigens and antibodies meet they combine to form an insoluble substance which may be ingested and then destroyed by the white cells in the blood. If sufficient white cells are available the disease is overcome and the victim is left with antibodies which may confer a degree of immunity from future attacks of the same micro-organism. Immunity may last for life, as with many childhood illnesses, or only for a few months, as with viruses such as those responsible for the common cold and for influenza, which mutate very rapidly.

This natural process is the basis of vaccination, and, nowadays, of innoculation, by a range of vaccines each prepared to give immunity from a specific disease with as little upset as possible. Vaccines are produced from the appropriate micro-organisms by processes that remove their toxic effects, and the dose is precisely controlled. Immunisation now gives protection to children against measles, whooping cough, diphtheria, poliomyelitis, tetanus, tuberculosis and German measles, and, to children and adults who travel abroad, against cholera, smallpox, typhoid and para-typhoid fevers, and yellow fever. The area physician responsible for schools will advise teachers who propose to take children abroad. The spectacular success of immunisation, especially against diphtheria and poliomyelitis, is shown in Table IV, Chapter 1. Such successes do not eliminate the micro-organisms, but limit their growth rate and reduce the reservoir of infection in the community.

The antibody reaction is not confined to pathogens: any foreign proteins, not merely those of invading micro-organisms, automatically cause the production of antibodies which attack them. Thus an implanted organ (such as a heart) is probably rejected unless the cells which produce antibodies are put out of action by drugs, thus destroying the body's defences and leaving it highly vulnerable to infection. This is why immunology is still a rapidly expanding field of biochemical research, despite its already great success in producing many vaccines.

Some of the measures adopted collectively in various parts of the world at different times to control communicable diseases were mentioned in Chapter 1. Successive governments have enacted a wide body of legislation. Some diseases (see Table IV) must be notified to the area medical officer, who is thus able to watch their incidence in his area and to take action when necessary. Area health authorities are empowered to make other diseases temporarily notifiable. This may be done in localised epidemics or, rarely today, when two clinically similar diseases (such as chickenpox and smallpox) are present. Other examples of measures enacted in national legislation include the provision of safe water, sewage disposal, food hygiene and safety, milk pasteurisation, rodent control, port health inspections, and control on imports of animals and animal products. International action, including the compilation of comprehensive statistics of the incidence of diseases, is undertaken by the World Health Organisation. These statistics, with others collected locally and nationally, form the basis of epidemiology.

Enough has been written to indicate how epidemics may begin, why they spread, why they die out and why, as for example with measles, they are often periodic. The reader may find it interesting to invent a disease-producing micro-organism with specified characteristics (such as its possible ways of being transmitted, the period of immunity the disease naturally confers on its victims, and the incubation period of the disease) and to attempt to make an approximate model of the resulting epidemic if the micro-organism makes its appearance in human carriers on Waterloo Station or on Dartmoor. It is easy to discover that an epidemic is not inevitable, but must depend on the number of carriers in relation to the number of potential hosts who are not immune from it—which in turn depends on when the disease made its previous appearance. And it is not difficult to estimate the shape of the curve which shows the number of cases at intervals since the epidemic began. Mathematical models of epidemics have been described by Kendall and others (see references).

This brief and in parts over-simplified account of the causes and characteristics of communicable diseases includes enough information to make the principles of personal and public hygiene meaningful to boys and girls. It also prompts the questions: What are the observations and experiments which justify at least some of the *ex cathedra* statements in the chapter? What special techniques must be employed? To what extent is it practicable or desirable to attempt such experiments in schools? A basic course of experimental microbiology (bacteriology) may well lead to an understanding that microbes exist in profusion and in great variety; that they can sometimes be recognised from their effects; that some conditions promote their rapid reproduction while others inhibit the growth of colonies or may kill the organisms; that most bacteria are harmless or beneficent. A properly organised course will teach the pupils how to handle bacteria safely, how to maintain sterile conditions and how correctly to dispose of contaminated materials.

A Microbiology in School Advisory Committee representing a range of microbiological and educational interests has recently been set up (MISAC—see references). The variety of organisms available to schools from biological suppliers has increased. Micro-organisms are also cultivated from a variety of habitats in schools such as the pupils themselves, cloakrooms, animal cages, and kitchens. Such cultures will almost certainly include some which are potentially pathogenic in man. This places on teachers a vital responsibility to insist on safety rules, on correct procedures in handling and disposing of cultures, and on discipline in the laboratory. The only safe rule is to assume that every culture is potentially dangerous, a rule which, in view of the probability of mutation and the known variation of human beings susceptibility to infection, is no more than common prudence. Essential precautions are contained in *The use of micro-organisms in schools* and in a number of other books—see references below. Notes on the commoner communicable diseases are in Appendix I.

References

Memorandum on the control of infectious diseases in schools, DES/DHSS, 1971.

Recommended practice for schools relating to the use of living organisms and material of living origin, Schools Council, EUP, 1974.

Keeping animals in schools, DES, HMSO, 1972.

Safety in science laboratories (2nd edition), DES, HMSO, 1976.

'Infectious Diseases', Ch. 7 in *The health of the school child* 1971–2, DES, HMSO, 1974.

'Review of Practical Manuals of Value to School Teachers Using Micro-organisms', in *Journal of biological education*, pp 331–337 vol. 5, No. 6, Institute of Biology, Institute of Biology, December, 1971.

The role of immunisation in communicable disease control (Public Health Papers, No. 8), WHO, 1961.

'Mathematical Models of the Spread of an Infection', in *Mathematics and computer science in biology and medicine*, D G Kendall, H.M.S.O, 1965.

'Micro-biology in Schools Advisory Committee' (MISAC) *Journal Biol. Ed.* 6, 207–210, B W Bainbridge, Institute of Biology, June, 1972.

The use of micro-organisms in schools, DES, HMSO, 1977.

Further reading

Man against disease (Biology Text 2), Nuffield Foundation, Longmans/ Penguin, 1966.

Health and hygiene (Combined Science Theme 3), Nuffield Foundation, Longmans, 1971.

War against Disease Book 7 in series Biology for the Individual, D Reid and P Booth, Heinemann, 1974.

The microbe hunters, P de Kruif, Harcourt, Brace (New York), 1932.

Antony van Leeuwenhoek and his little animals, C Dobell (Ed.), Dever (U.S.) 1932.

'Epidemics of endemic disease', Ch. 14 in *The natural history of infectious diseases* (4th edition), Sir F Macfarlane Burnet, CUP, 1972.

Man, nature, and disease, R Fiennes, Weidenfeld and Nicolson, 1964.

King cholera: the biography of a disease, N Longmate, Hamish Hamilton, 1966

'Infection', Ch. 6 in *Biology, man, and society*, A Cornwell, McGraw Hill, 1974.

Human health, biology and hygiene, D T D Hughes and P T Marshall, CUP, 1970.

Chapters 1–20 in *Man against disease*, A G Clegg and P C Clegg, Heinemann, 1973.

*Bacterial food poisoning, J Taylor (Ed.), Royal Society of Health, 1969.

*Biological defence mechanisms, I Carr, Blackwell, 1972.

*'Medical Aspects of Biochemistry' Ch. 8 in *Biochemistry–a special study* (Advanced Science—Chemistry), Nuffield Foundation, Penguin, 1970.

*'Models for Infectious Diseases', Ch. 11 in *Data handling in epidemiology*, H V Mumsam: W W Holland (Ed.), OUP, 1970.

6

POLLUTION

Pollution has been defined as 'the presence of toxic materials introduced into our environment by man' (K Mellanby—see references), to which may be added disturbing effects such as excessive noise. So pollution concerns the surface of the land, which may be spoiled by industrial waste and by litter; water, which may be fouled by toxic solutes and by sewage; and the atmosphere, which may contain smoke and other irritants as well as sound waves of sufficient energy to cause discomfort or even deafness. Although pollutants are invariably a nuisance in reducing amenity they also sometimes endanger health, so consideration of them is part of health education. A more detailed discussion of the occupational dangers associated with work with various toxic substances is in Chapter 7. Here we shall review briefly certain general aspects of pollution as they affect the community as a whole, and then consider three specific examples.

When technology is applied to industry, including agriculture and transport, the first order effect may nowadays be assumed to benefit society. But there are also almost invariably what Lord Ashby (see reference) has described as second order effects which may not always have been foreseen (or may not even have been foreseeable at the time) and which do not benefit the community. These effects constitute pollution. Pollution is at its worst where intensive technological use of natural resources takes place in densely populated areas. Some of the more obvious kinds of pollution, such as smoke from coal burning, are legacies of the past when little regard was paid to the welfare of the majority. One of the most interesting features of present day industrial societies is their increasing willingness to allow their law makers to abate pollution in the knowledge that such steps will put up the cost of many products they wish to enjoy. Lord Justice Thesiger's opinion, uttered in 1879, that what would be a nuisance in Belgrave Square would not necessarily be so in Bermondsey, would arouse little sympathy today.

Other forms of pollution can arise as unsuspected second order effects, for instance the effects of pesticides, which are intended to increase the production of crops and livestock in an increasingly hungry world by reducing the loss—estimated at some £300 million a year in Britain alone—due to pests of crops and insect damage to farm stock. This they do, but they create new problems as well.

Hazards to health have originated directly or indirectly (through food and water) from the use of hormones to increase meat production and the use of fertilisers to increase the yield of crops. It is important to know what happens to pesticides or, indeed, to any potentially dangerous substances after they are used or released. Some, such as the weedkiller paraquat, a deadly poison if taken by man, are soon rendered harmless by contact with the soil. Others, such as the hormone herbicide 2:4–D persist and therefore contaminate the soil for years. A particularly serious hazard occurs where a toxic substance accumulates in living organisms, which most often happens in water. Contaminated fish then present a hazard to predators, including man. The fate of the 41 Japanese who died from mercury poisoning after eating fish taken from Minimata Bay offers a well-documented warning of such dangers, fortunately rare.

Despite the view expressed earlier that in general industrial communities often accept the cost of reducing or eliminating pollution, there are some causes, which can be readily identified, and where remedies are known, for which the financial cost of the cure is more than those responsible will willingly accept. An extreme example could arise, for example, in the case of an airport which can present the surrounding community with the choice of unemployment if it has to close down or with putting up with pollution if the enterprise is to stay in business. There is also the difficulty of the legacy of pollution caused by organisations which no longer exist. The main difficulty is, as stated in the *First report of the Royal Commission on environmental pollution* (1971), that pollution's main economic characteristic is that its costs are not usually borne by the polluters, so that production may be pushed beyond the point which is best for society. The need then arises for some means of arbitration which takes into account the relationship between different scales of value, economic on the one hand and social on the other.

Control operates at two levels. First, there is potential control at the individual and group levels. Individuals can do a great deal voluntarily, for instance, by not incinerating garden rubbish and by exhorting their neighbours not to do so. Groups of individuals have been successful in eliminating a local threat of noise pollution from airfields and motorways, sometimes by causing the nuisance to be transferred elsewhere. Schools have contributed by removing rubbish from streams and in improving industrial waste dumps. Some groups exert influence through the publicity media, and provoke constructive discussion, or sometimes violent controversy.

Secondly, there is control at local government, central government and international levels. Local authorities are responsible for amenity and health in their areas. They have considerable powers, for instance in establishing smoke-control areas and monitoring levels of local air pollution. Central government can and does act through legislation, such as the Alkali Act of 1863 prompted by acid emissions from the manufacture of alkalis, and the Clean Air Acts of 1956 and 1968, for which the London smog of 1952 undoubtedly acted as a stimulus.

Central governing also provides and maintains the public health laboratory service and conducts, or appoints other organisations to conduct, research. Examples of such bodies are the Water Pollution Research Laboratory at Stevenage, the Air Pollution Research Unit of the Medical Research Council, and the Water Resources Board which co-ordinates the work of the river authorities and reports directly to central government. Many problems, however, concern two or more nations—for example, some air pollution in Scandinavia comes from Britain, while Holland suffers pollution of the Rhine from Germany— but the potential for international control exists through World Health Organisation.

We now consider in some detail three examples of pollution.

a. Air Pollution

Significant pollution of the air above the larger towns of Britain dates from the thirteenth century which saw the beginning of the widespread use of coal. In 1306 Parliament decreed that the use of coal in lime burning just outside the boundary of the City of London be banned, and the first offender was executed soon afterwards. More recently the Clean Air Acts of 1956 and 1968 enabled local authorities to prohibit the emission of smoke from domestic fires and gave greater powers both to local authorities and to government officials to control emissions of grit, dust and smoke from industrial plant. The results can be seen in many industrial cities, large areas of which now enjoy comparatively clean air. In London it has been estimated that winter sunshine has increased by a half as a direct consequence of the legislation of 1956.

Air pollution is caused by gases (mainly carbon monoxide, the oxides of sulphur and nitrogen, and hydrocarbons), and by solid or liquid particles such as smoke (carbon), grit, liquid hydrocarbons and solutes of organic compounds, and by acids such as hydrochloric and sulphuric.

Globally carbon monoxide is the most abundant polluting gas. It is usually present in air at a background concentration of 0·1 of a part per million, but has on occasion attained 300 parts per million in London. Exposure for an hour or two to a concentration of 100 parts per million can reduce the oxygen content of the blood sufficiently to cause dizziness and headache, related usually to a 15 per cent saturation of carboxy-haemoglobin in the blood. About 11,000 million kilograms of carbon monoxide are released annually into the skies of Britain, mainly from the exhausts of motor vehicles. But fortunately, although concentrations may occasionally reach a high level in heavy traffic or in road tunnels the gas, being about as dense as air, disperses quickly: although chemically stable (except possibly at the top of the troposphere), the background concentration, despite increasing emission, has remained virtually constant for 25 years. The reservoir of carbon monoxide is kept under control by scavengers, which are probably micro-organisms in the soil which convert carbon monoxide into methane—another example of beneficent microbes. So the carbon monoxide level in the air does not present an acute problem: in fact more carbon monoxide is absorbed in the blood as a result of cigarette smoking than from breathing air in a busy street. It has often been pointed out that a policeman who smokes cigarettes is better protected from carbon monoxide poisoning when he is on point duty in the heaviest traffic, because he cannot then smoke, than when he is at home.

Sulphur dioxide is a very important gaseous pollutant in the air over Britain (about 6,000 million kilograms annually) mainly as a consequence of power generation. A concentration of 0·2 of a part per million for three days causes respiratory troubles in animals and a concentration of half of this results in damage to crops such as wheat and apples. Urban concentrations still sometimes exceed this level. The London smog of 1952 gave an average of 1·34 parts per million over a period of two days.

Some observers (see, for example, *Pollution in the year 2000* by K Mellanby) believe that, after sulphur dioxide, fluoride emissions are the most dangerous forms of air pollution in the United Kingdom. They occur both as a gas, hydrogen fluoride, and as minute particles of compounds of fluorine. They come from brickworks, steelworks, fertiliser manufacture and from the smelting of aluminium. The Alkali Inspectorate controls discharges by specifying a maximum concentration in the atmosphere and a maximum ground level concentration. The total quantity is relatively small, but hydrofluoric acid is so poisonous that the maximum allowed concentration is very low. Extremely small concentrations can affect plants. For example, according to data published in the United States, ·005 of a part per million at ground level will blight maize, and ·001 of a part per million is said to lower citrus fruit production. The average fluoride content of herbage in the United Kingdom is five parts per million, which is far larger than the tolerable level of fluorine compounds in the air. If grazing land is exposed continuously to an air concentration of hydrogen fluoride greater than 1 microgram per cubic metre the level of fluoride in herbage may reach a concentration of 30–35 parts per million, when dairy cows are considered to be at risk and may suffer a range of illnesses from loss of teeth to lameness. So the siting of, for example, a brickworks in the countryside needs care. The sources of fluoride in the diet, including atmospheric pollution, were discussed by Dr A E Martin in a paper presented to the Health Congress of the Royal Society of Health in 1971 (see references).

Particle pollution in the air has the effect of cutting down natural daylight by absorption of some of the frequencies in sunlight, and also causes the deposition of dirt, to the extent of about one kilogram of solid materials falling annually on each square metre in heavy industrial areas. Much of this dirt is ash and soot from the combustion of coal and oil but specific industries, such as cement and steel, make their own contributions. The particles range in diameter from about ·001 to 1000 micrometres but most are in the range 0·1 to 10 micrometres. Particles smaller than 0·07 micrometres are susceptible to Brownian motion and thus remain suspended in the atmosphere and contribute to haze. Some haze is attributable to oxides of nitrogen and to unburnt hydrocarbons from vehicle exhausts, which is one of several reasons for the control of exhaust emission in the United States, where the prevalence in some areas of inversions of air temperature in anticyclonic conditions aggravates the nuisance. Exhaust from internal combustion engines also includes aldehydes and varying quantities of lead, which, as tetra ethyl lead, is a fuel additive for petrol engines with a high compression ratio.

b. Pesticides
Pesticides are intended to destroy organisms which attack the plants and animals which man uses for food. It is beyond dispute that the present population of the world, let alone future increases, cannot exist if man's competitors are not kept within reasonable bounds. The difficulty lies in isolating a substance which eliminates the particular pest but not the domesticated plants or animals, or the subsequent human consumer. It is difficult, too, to ensure that the pesticide is applied only to its target. For instance seed dressings, frequently containing mercury compounds, are intended to control the fungal parasites of the crops. They sometimes kill birds which eat the seeds—birds which can be regarded by the farmer as parasites or by the conservationist as desirable species at risk. The important point is the effect on the whole biosphere, of which man and bird are part, if all the birds were destroyed.

Hormone herbicides are synthetic compounds which resemble the natural hormones of susceptible broad-leaved weeds sufficiently closely to produce lethal abnormalities while leaving grain crops relatively unharmed. The herbicide 4-chloro-2 methylphenoxyacetic acid (MCPA) is a modern example. This selective weedkiller can of course cause damage to broad-leaved crops and natural flora by careless spraying or through changes of wind direction. As distinct from some of its precursors this herbicide does not persist appreciably in the soil.

The organochlorine compound DDT began to be used in the 1939–45 war to control malaria and typhus by eliminating the insects which spread these diseases. Widespread use has since resulted in a great deal of contamination of animals, especially in aquatic habitats. This is a very clear example of a second order effect, unfortunate but probably of less significance than the first order effect for which this efficient insecticide was originally produced. None the less it has caused the use of DDT to be banned in some parts of the world—an illustration of the influence of pressure groups.

c. Synthetic Detergents
The virtual replacement of soap (except for personal hygiene) by syn-

thetic detergents in the past few years is an interesting example both of useful domestic technology with unsuspected second order effects, and of the steps which have been taken to reduce some of those effects. There are three second order effects. The first is that about three times as much energy is needed to make these detergents as to make equivalently effective quantities of soap. The second is that when first produced they were not bio-degradable. (Soap is bio-degradable: microbes break it down to carbon dioxide and water.) So foam from synthetic detergents persisted in the sewage farm and interfered with its processes, and persisted in the rivers where it was often sufficient to reduce the uptake of oxygen by the water to the extent that fish died in large numbers. The third second order effect is that the phosphates from detergents may disturb the biological cycle in some lakes and rivers. When nitrates (which may come from fertilisers) and phosphates are freely available in soil water the growth of algae and other forms of plant life in lakes and rivers may increase very rapidly because of an over-abundance of these nutrients. In consequence lakes and reservoirs in particular may become covered with algae so that the lower layers of the water are in shadow, and plants cannot flourish. The algae die and decompose, further deoxygenising the water. This is probable only in lowland lakes, in reservoirs, and in slow moving rivers and is therefore not a serious problem in this country, but it has become so in parts of the United States and Canada. As the second and third of these side effects began to be observed there was widespread unease leading to the setting up (in 1957) of a Standing Technical Committee on Synthetic Detergents. This Committee pressed manufacturers to seek a material which would be broken down at the sewage works or in the river, and by 1959 such a degradable compound was synthetised, but it cost more than the original wetting agent and needed additional capital investment for manufacture. The Committee then organised trials of the new detergents, via secretly arranged sale in two towns, where the effects on both the sewage works and the river, and the effects, if any, on unsuspecting housewives, could be monitored. The trials were sufficiently conclusive to enable the Committee to secure a voluntary undertaking from the manufacturers to phase out the non-degradable wetting agents as soon as the newer form could be produced. So, by voluntary co-operation, the objectionable second order effect of foaming has been practically eliminated. But in the United States and Canada the problem has not been so happily resolved.

These three examples of pollution have been described superficially, but it is hoped in sufficient detail to illustrate several useful teaching points.

First there is the truism, which is sometimes overlooked, that although these topics demand good judgement, no judgement, and no useful discussion, is possible without knowledge. The knowledge required for a full understanding of these examples includes absorption of sunlight by the atmosphere; some of the properties of carbon monoxide, sulphur, nitrogen, and oxygen; the meaning of words or phrases such as hydrocarbons, organic compounds, concentration, density, chemical stability, the troposphere, Brownian motion, inversions and anticyclones, compression ratios, pests, fungal parasites, hormones, energy, and substances which are degradable by microbes; as well as several geographical facts and related ideas such as fast moving air streams and prevailing winds; some understanding of economics. This knowledge is acquired only gradually by boys and girls as a result of studying several disciplines, and many of them are clarified only when pupils have had the benefit of a range of experiences in the laboratory, in the field and in the library.

Secondly, there is the fact that the consequences of an apparently simple action (such as changing the kind of cleaning agents bought by housewives) may be unforeseeable, will almost certainly not all be foreseen, and may be very considerable. Some of these consequences may appear to be marginal but very slight changes in local conditions, such as the rate of flow of a river, can alter the ecological balance from safe disposal to major pollution.

Thirdly, we must appreciate that the causes of chronic illness are rarely simple. It would be tempting, for example, to correlate the incidence of bronchitis with the level of sulphur dioxide in the air, but misleading to do so because sulphur dioxide is rarely found alone as a pollutant and the causes of bronchitis are many.

Fourthly, the examples illustrate the growth of what Lord Ashby described in his lecture already referred to as 'social feedback', leading to the abatement of pollution by law or by consent as soon as the pollutant becomes a nuisance.

Fifthly, we see that 'social feedback' begins with individuals. The beginnings of understanding about pollution should occur in early childhood. Despite the formidable technical vocabulary listed under the first point there is much, even at the simple level of encouraging children not to litter the countryside, which is the responsibility of parents and of infant and primary school teachers to convey. Notions of the interdependence of living things can be introduced at an early age.

Sixthly, we can learn that a sense of proportion is more helpful than an hysterical reaction to the latest 'doomwatch' scare. Deaths and illness directly attributable to types of pollution discussed in this chapter are trivial in number compared with those caused by cigarette smoke, by far the most dangerous form of air pollution; and by accidents, which ought perhaps to be regarded as another form of pollution. The main stimuli for 'social feedback' are the need to preserve, if not improve, amenity, and the view that 'where there's muck there's money' is no longer acceptable. The effects of a given pollutant are likely to vary widely from individual to individual, and appreciation of this fact (with a sense of proportion) involves the acceptance of ideas of variation and probability.

A study of pollution, or of conservation, is often included in general studies in the sixth form and in courses of social biology in schools and elsewhere. Some of the topics included in this chapter lend themselves to experimental work which is practicable in secondary schools. Several examples are described by K Mellanby in *The biology of pollution* (see references).

References

The biology of pollution (Institute of Biology 'Studies in Biology'—No. 38), K Mellanby, Edward Arnold. 1972.

Pesticides and pollution, K Mellanby, Collins, 1969.

Report of the Royal Commission on Environmental Pollution, Royal Commission, HMSO, September, 1971.

'Air Pollution' in *Endeavour* vol. 30 pp, 107–114, R A Papetti and F R Gilmore, Pergamon, 1971.

'Prospect for Pollution', in *Community health*, vol. 5, No. 2, pp 92–100, Lord Ashby, John Wright and Sons, September/October, 1973.

Air pollution and its effects on food production and contamination (Congress Report), Dr A E Martin, Royal Society of Health, 1971.

Further reading

'Water', (Sec. 6) 'Food and Land', (Sec. 3) 'Air', (Sec. 8) and Appendix 4 in *Maintaining the environment* (course units 26 and 27), The Open University Technology Foundation, The Open University Press.

'Air', (Ch. 1) 'Water', (Ch. 2) 'Soil', (Ch. 4) in *Health hazards of the human environment* (prepared by 100 specialists in 15 countries), WHO, 1972.

*'Cancer and Bronchitis Mortality in Relation to Atmospheric Deposits and Smoke', in *British Medical Journal*, vol. 1, No. 5114, pp 74–79, P Stocks, BMA, 1959.

7

SOME DANGERS ARISING FROM THE USE OF TOXIC MATERIALS IN INDUSTRY

The association of certain illnesses with industrial jobs has been recognised for many years. Silicosis; necrosis of the jaw ('phossy jaw' which used to accompany the manufacture of early types of matches in which white phosphorus was used); and the phrase 'as mad as a hatter' (from the occurrence of mercury poisoning in the hatting trade when mercuric nitrate was used to cure the felt) are reminders of such occupational risks. The great increase in industrial processes in the last half century has caused many other occupational hazards gradually to be recognised, and increasingly contained by a combination of industrial medicine, codes of practice (sometimes mandatory), improved methods for the detection of toxic substances in small concentrations, the extraction of dust from factory areas and the wearing of means of protection. Some dangers are significant only when there is frequent exposure to a toxic material, but there is growing evidence that infrequent or slight exposure to many substances may also be dangerous. Poisonous substances can and do find their way into the atmosphere, the soil, and into water supplies, and become potential or actual hazards to the community at large. The disposal of industrial waste now demands and receives close attention.

The Factories Act 1961 sets out the legal requirements in respect of atmospheric pollution by factories. The Deposit of Poisonous Waste Act 1972 requires that poisonous, noxious or polluting waste shall not be deposited on land or water so as to give rise to environmental hazard. The Health and Safety at Work etc Act 1974 requires that the health, safety and welfare of all persons shall be protected against hazards which may exist as a result of the activities of those at work.

HM Factory Inspectorate, Health and Safety Executive, issues Technical Data Notes which set out the limits below which there is considered to be no significant threat to health, and the safety precautions to be taken in respect of over 500 substances.

Regulations to be made under various sections of the Health and Safety at Work etc Act 1974 and Section 2(2) of the European Communities Act 1972 (b) are in draft form and to date indicate the nature and level of the risks involved and the precautions to be taken in the handling of 1,090 substances.

Public health workers now distinguish between monitoring and surveillance. Monitoring refers to the making of routine observations on the health of individuals and on factors in the environment such as the concentration of lead, while surveillance is the process of collating and interpreting the data obtained from monitoring programmes with the objective of detecting changes in health patterns in populations. Surveillance is made increasingly feasible by the development of techniques for data handling. But in practice establishing a correlation between a factor in the environment and health trends is a difficult and long-term process, because the number of variables, including variations in human susceptibility, is large, and the development of diseases, such as some forms of cancer, may be slow. This is why it has taken many years to appreciate the potential dangers of substances which used to be considered safe.

This is why, when there are grounds for suspicion which fall short of proof, we look for safer alternatives, or substances against whose harmful effects it is easier to protect ourselves; and, above all, take all reasonable precautions in the use of the suspected substance. In other words, we should reduce to a minimum the amount of exposure and take every precaution against inhalation, ingestion or absorption of the substance. However dangerous a substance is, it can only actually do harm when it gets into the body—through the nose, mouth or skin. Even then our bodies have their own defence mechanisms which in one way or another can either change many potentially harmful substances into relatively or absolutely harmless ones, or can excrete them before they have had time to do serious harm. But there is a point beyond which these defence mechanisms do not operate, and that point varies from person to person; it differs with age and with the general state of health, among other variables.

We shall now consider as examples lead, mercury, asbestos and radioactive substances. All occur naturally and all have been put to widespread use in the service of man; lead and mercury since prehistoric times, asbestos more recently, and radioactive substances only in this century. As we have become more aware of the hazards associated with their use measures have been introduced which, while still allowing us to use them for purposes which we regard as essential or desirable, increasingly reduce the risks we take when using them. One obvious measure is to reduce the amount we use as far as possible and then to ensure that we reduce the chances of getting them inside our bodies to the absolute minimum. This is important for all of us, but particularly for children. By taking sensible precautions (use sparingly and take care) we can use these substances in schools with reasonable certainty that no pupil will, as a result of such use, suffer any of the consequences described below.

Lead

The dangers of industrial poisoning have been known since the last century when lead was widely used in the manufacture of paint and for glazes in the pottery trade. The steps nowadays taken to minimise the dangers to industrial workers are described in Technical Data Note 16 *The prevention of industrial lead poisoning* and in a Code of Practice (see references). The Factories Act 1961 includes several sections of legislation to protect those who work with lead. Lead may enter the body by both ingestion and, in the form of dust or fumes, by inhalation. Whether in the form of metallic lead or of a compound, lead ions, either present in the substance or formed within the body, are absorbed in the bone and accumulate there. These are gradually released into the system and can have the effect in adults of causing undue fatigue, constipation, disturbed sleep, and in time, harm to the central nervous system. These effects are heightened in children and young people, who may suffer severe brain damage which shows itself in irritability and irrational behaviour. Some expert opinion asserts that lead poisoning may be a factor in mental retardation of children. For this reason people under the age of 18 are banned from some lead-using industrial processes.

As well as in industry, lead and its compounds can be found in many commonly used materials such as paints, pottery glazes, water-pipes and petrol. A greater awareness of the dangers of lead poisoning has resulted in the replacement of lead water-pipes with the copper type in soft-water areas, and a reduction in the lead content of petrol. But there are many simple precautions that can be taken to reduce further the hazards of using lead-based materials, of which personal hygiene is, as when any dangerous substance is handled, of major importance.

The mandatory precautions to be observed when using lead include: lead paint in the form of a spray may not be used in the interior painting of buildings; non-lead materials like titanium oxide must be substituted for white lead in paint manufacture; lead should not be rubbed down except by wet techniques. It is also essential to limit the dust-producing stages of some processes by enclosing them and removing the dust by exhaust ventilation.

The other precautions include cleanliness of lavatories and washrooms, strict attention to personal hygiene and the provision of special protective clothing, instructions to workers, notification to HM Chief Inspector of Factories when it is believed that a patient is suffering from lead poisoning contracted in any factory, and periodic medical examination of persons employed in processes using lead. It is nowadays possible to detect lead absorption in the body long before the stage of clinical lead poisoning.

Mercury
Mercury has a higher vapour pressure than lead at ordinary temperatures. If mercury is exposed in a closed room at normal temperatures the concentration of mercury vapour may rise to more than 100 times the threshold limit value. Like lead, mercury has a range of inorganic

and organic compounds which to a greater or less extent are toxic. Technical Data Note (21) *Mercury* (see references) summarises the toxic effects and precautions needed in industry.

In brief, prolonged exposure to the metal mercury, its oxides and metallic salts may produce chronic poisoning. Early symptoms may include nausea, headache, tiredness and chronic diarrhoea, with possible excessive salivation, bleeding from the gums, ulceration and loosening of teeth. Muscular tremors appear early; psychic disturbance appears as abnormal shyness, loss of confidence, irritability, vague fears and depression and even loss of memory, hallucinations or mental deterioration. Toxic organo-mercury compounds, on the other hand, have more pronounced effects on the central nervous system and may produce tremors, loss of co-ordination, difficulty in speaking clearly, and constriction of the visual fields.

Methods of control in industry include strict attention to cleanliness in work places, with benches designed so that no droplets can collect in cracks or crevices. Mercury is stored in air-tight or water-sealed vessels. Spillage must be removed immediately. Processes are fully enclosed wherever possible. When this is not possible the maximum degree of enclosure is supported by exhaust ventilation. Personal protection includes protective clothing, breathing apparatus for emergency use, and a very high standard of washing facilities. Eating and drinking are forbidden in workrooms.

The most probable cause of danger from mercury poisoning in the environment in general, as opposed to the factory, arises from some organo-mercury compounds. There is evidence that in some circumstances inorganic mercury can be made to react with organic materials to produce methyl mercury by the action of micro-organisms. Methyl mercury can enter food chains through uptake by aquatic plants, algae, low forms of animal life, and fish, in which the concentration may be high. The first major report of mercury poisoning from industrial waste in the Minamata Bay area of Japan was referred to in the previous chapter. This disaster was caused by methyl mercury, a waste product of an acetaldehyde manufacturing process in which a mercury catalyst is used, which although present in the water at an undetectably low level was greatly concentrated by fish and shell fish which took it up.

Various mercury compounds have been used to treat seed potatoes, flower bulbs and grain seeds in several parts of the world, and several consequent cases of poisoning have recently been reported, including an incident in Iraq in 1972 causing more than 200 deaths.

These two metals, among others, are naturally occurring toxic substances with toxic derivatives which are inevitably present at a low background concentration taken up in minute quantities by everyone. Great care is taken to protect those who work with lead or mercury, but the possibility of local high concentrations—sufficient to cause very unpleasant illnesses—has to be continually watched for. Recent studies of the distribution and effects of these elements are reported in *Health hazards of the human environment* (see references).

Asbestos

A useful summary of the present state of knowledge about asbestos is contained in *Asbestos, health hazards and precautions* (see references).

It was not until the 1920s that the hazards to health of heavy exposure to asbestos were first suspected, and quickly confirmed. Later still its carcinogenic potential was recognised. It is not surprising therefore that all the firm knowledge we have is about situations of greatest risk, namely, occupational exposure. Little if anything is known at present about the possible connection between ill-health and the presence of asbestos dust in the general environment. In the meantime it is prudent to assume that we do accept some degree of risk in using asbestos, and to reduce that risk by avoiding as far as we possibly can any addition to the asbestos dust in the atmosphere.

Radioactive Substances

Radioactive substances of various origins are rather different and very widely discussed sources of potential danger to workers in the appropriate fields and, in some circumstances, to a wider public. Teachers who are permitted to use radioactive substances in schools are subject to restrictions (stated in Administrative Memorandum 2/76 (DES)) which are based on very careful analysis of data obtained from exposure of both human beings and animals. Those who are interested in the evidence on which safety precautions for the use of radioactive materials and other sources of ionising radiations are based may refer to various books mentioned at the end of this chapter. Here it is sufficient to point out that the maximum permissible dose of radiation has been reduced several times as knowledge of the dangerous effects has accumulated. Even so the present level does not ensure that no one will be harmed, but the risks are considered sufficiently small in comparison with the benefits to the community and, compared with other risks to health, reasonable and acceptable. Although much higher doses are administered to patients for diagnostic and therapeutic purposes, improvements in techniques are constantly being sought so as to reduce the dose required.

Hygiene was regarded in Chapter 5 as a matter of limiting the distribution of micro-organisms which cause disease—essentially a question of cleanliness. It requires ever-increasing foresight, vigilance and legislation in order to ensure that air, water and foodstuffs do not contain harmful ingredients.

References

Technical data notes: *Threshold limit values for* 1975 (Ref. 2/75), HM Factory Inspectorate, Dept. of Employment, 1976 (Annual).

Prevention of industrial lead poisoning. (16) (2nd Edition), 1975.

Mercury (21) (2nd Edition), 1973.

Control of asbestos dust (35), 1972.

Standards for asbestos dust concentration for use with Asbestos Regulations, 1969 (13) (2nd Edition), 1974.

Health: dust in industry (14), 1970.

Lead: health precautions, HSE, 1976.

Problems arising from the use of asbestos, Dept. of Employment, HMSO, 1968.

Asbestos and you, HSE, Employment Medical Advisory Service, 1975.

Asbestos: health hazards and precautions (an interim statement by the Advisory Committee on Asbestos), Health and Safety Commission, HMSO, 1977.

'Radiation', Ch. 5 in *The biology of pollution* (Institute of Biology: Studies in Biology No. 38), K Mellanby, Edward Arnold, 1972.

'Asbestos Wool' (para. 71) 'Carcinogenic substances' (paras 93, 94A) 'Lead' (para. 107B) 'Mercury' (para. 108A) 'Ionising Radiations' (paras. 76, 140, 141, 142.) all in DES Safety Series No. 2, Second edition, *Safety in science laboratories,* DES, HMSO, 1976.

The use of asbestos in educational establishments. Administrative Memorandum 7/76 (5/76 Welsh Office), DES and Welsh Office, 1976.

Further reading

'Environmental Hazards from Ionising Radiation', Chapter 9 in *Maintaining the Environment* (Course units 2 and 26), Open University Technology Foundation, Open University Press, 1972.

Biological effects of radiation (The Wykcham Science Series), J E Coggle and G R Noakes, Wykeham Publications, 1971.

Radiation and health (monitoring processes in air and water), The Royal Society of Health, 1971.

'Lead, Mercury, Asbestos'; Ch. 12 'Ionising Radiation'; Ch. 14, in *Health hazards of the human environment,* WHO, HMSO, 1973.

Radiochemical manual, United Kingdom Atomic Energy Authority: Radiochemical Centre, 1966.

8

ACCIDENTS

The World Health Organisation has defined an accident as an unpremeditated event resulting in a recognisable injury.

The Registrar General's Statistical Review (1971) shows that in England and Wales, in each of the years from 1961 until 1971, approximately 19,000 people died as the result of accidents. The annual number of deaths from the main sources of accidents, which vary somewhat from year to year, averaged approximately as follows:

transport of all kinds	7,700
of which road traffic accidents accounted for	7,000
falls	5,500
poisons, including gases and vapours	850
fire	700
drowning	600

These causes account for more than three-quarters of the total.

Another way of looking at the statistics is to divide accidents into categories based on the type of location—for example, those occurring in travelling, at work, and in the home. This shows rather more than 7,000 deaths occurring in the home (including many of the deaths due to falls, poison and fire), and about 750 in factories or coal mines or on farms. The number of deaths due to accidents in the home year by year slightly exceeds the number of deaths due to road accidents.

But death is not the most usual result of an accident. The number of serious injuries, by which are meant injuries often necessitating a stay in hospital, such as fractures, concussion, internal injuries, crushing, severe cuts and lacerations, and general shock requiring treatment, is approximately 90,000 a year on the roads and more than 100,000 in the home. About 250,000 injuries causing more than three days' absence from work are recorded annually in factories. The estimated annual total of all serious injuries, some of which are so severe as to lead to permanent disablement, is of the order of half a million. So the odds against an individual being killed or injured by accident in a given year are about 100 to 1. But this ratio is misleading. The distribution of casualties among various kinds of accidents is markedly different from age group to age group, and between the sexes—for example, boys and men are much more liable to road accidents than girls and women, while women are (not surprisingly) more vulnerable than men in the home.

Chance, or 'bad luck', does not cause accidents. But chance, or a chance combination of circumstances, may decide whether or not an accident will follow an act of human carelessness, or whether a natural event such as a lightning flash results in an accident to someone. Chance, or circumstances beyond the control of the victim, determines the severity of the result.

Accidents illustrate the suggestion in Chapter 1 that health (or ill health as a consequence of an accident) is determined by an interaction between the environment, the genetic constitution of the individual, and the behaviour both of individuals and of groups. In this sense the vital element in the environment may be for example a loose stair carpet, a frayed electric lead, a slippery road, a rotten rope, or a bicycle with defective brakes. The genetic constitution of the individual may determine his ability to react swiftly to emergency, his ability to visualise the possible consequences of carelessness and inattention, his ability to withstand fatigue, or his ability in some circumstances to control aggression and impatience. The behaviour of groups decides the acceptance or rejection of measures to protect others, such as the use of the breathalyser or the recommendations of a local fire officer. The behaviour of an individual, which may be affected by his genetic inheritance but not solely determined by it, is related to his attitude to safety in general and to his view of his responsibilities as an individual and, as a member of a group, towards other people. Morality cannot be excluded from a discussion of accidents and their prevention.

An accident-free technological world is not attainable, if only because human beings are liable to fatigue, illness, errors of judgement, and momentary lapses of concentration. The problem is how to minimise both the frequency of accidents and their consequences. The extent to which this can be done depends partly on cost, partly on education. If, for example, an aircraft crashes because of metal fatigue in a vital component, this is not an Act of God, but an act determined by the extent to which the community is willing to accept occasional disaster because of metal fatigue. Assuming a very high level of inspection of aircraft, which the community insists on, the only way further to reduce the risk of metal fatigue is to re-design and replace or to shorten the allowed operational life of the relevant metal components. So, to push the argument to absurdity, if every aircraft were replaced by a new one every week this particular danger would be negligible, but the cost would be unacceptable. The extent to which the environment can be made accident-proof is determined in part, but only in part, by cost. The other factors are knowledge and understanding. Cost is not likely to be so significant, but cannot always be ignored, in a vital domestic matter such as replacement of a broken electric mains outlet in the kitchen. The need here is to know enough to recognise the danger and to be able to cope with it—in other words for sound education, in this instance in home economics and in basic science.

On the human side the problem demands balance and judgement because gambling, or assessing risks, is a universal, and many would say, essential characteristic of human behaviour. No human actions are risk-free but some are much more hazardous than others. The educational problem is to balance the skill against the risk. Most would agree that it is better to accept the risks of motoring, crossing the road, sailing, climbing, cooking, pottery, playing darts, football, tennis, cricket, skiing, walking in the hills—in fact of living—than to forego them to avoid the risk of accident. In this kind of activity the teacher's job is to help the child to acquire the skill, and the confidence which comes only from knowledge and skill (which includes a realisation of an individual's limits of skill and of ability to assess risk), so that accidents are reduced to a minimum.

But accidents have been defined as certain unpremeditated events. Drowning because a dinghy capsizes in a sudden gust of wind should not be possible because the crew should be sufficiently skilled to foresee the possibility and judge the effect of the gust, and should have been educated to react correctly. Such an incident becomes an accident because of an educational failure. But if the dinghy was shattered by a shark in Southampton Water the incident would qualify as an accident because a teacher of sailing in England could not reasonably be expected to include in his course provision for this highly improbable event. On the other hand such an omission might well be regarded as a lapse in a sailing instructor in the Seychelles. Likewise if a boy determines to seduce a girl and succeeds, and she becomes pregnant, she cannot call it an accident (although she may well consider herself unlucky or unwise) since the boy's action was premeditated. He has not caused an accident; he has deliberately accepted the risk that his action may lead to the consequence of pregnancy.

During 1974, 14,697 children under the age of 15 died in England and Wales, 12,381 of them less than 5 years old. Of the total, 630 died as a result of motor vehicle accidents and 843 from all other accidents. Of those who died in motor vehicle accidents, 148 were under 5 years old and 482 (of whom 302 were boys) were between 5 and 14. In all other accidents, 537 children under 5 and 306 between 5 and 14, died. Most of the fatal accidents to children under 5 occurred in their homes. Deaths from all causes numbered 2,316 in the 5–14 age group, showing that about one third of all deaths in this group were caused by accidents. It is difficult to estimate the number of serious injuries, but a guess of at least 10 times as many as the number of fatalities on the roads is probably conservative. Some of these accidents result in most distressing permanent injuries.

It is not astonishing that the home is the most dangerous place for very young children because it is where they spend most of their time. Likewise the number of accidents to old people in the home is relatively very high. One of the most encouraging signs of care and consideration for others revealed by older boys and girls at school is the way in which groups of them have from time to time attempted successfully to devise domestic apparatus safe for old or handicapped people—a most helpful spin-off from the growing interest in technology and engineering design.

A survey in 1971 and 1972 (by the Medical Officer of Health and the Health Education Officer for Norwich—see references) of 910 children under 15 who had sustained accidents attended to at the casualty department of a local hospital showed that 678 (74–75 per cent) were under 5 years old. Boys were more prone to accidents than girls, and in preschool children the highest incidence was among the 2 to 3-year-olds of both sexes. There appeared to be no peak month when accidents were most frequent, and their incidence was not significantly high on any particular weekday. But the highest rate of accidents to children under 5 occurred between 9 am and noon—the time when mothers do the greater part of their routine work of the day and the children are likely to be most wide awake and active. In 95 per cent of the cases one or both parents were in charge at the time of the accident: in only six cases was a teenager in charge. No child was involved in an accident while left unattended in the house. There was no greater liability to accidents in 'one-parent' families.

The accident rates per 1,000 population (in the given age group) for 1972 were:

Age	no of accidents	size of population	rate per 1,000
0 – 4	405	8,825	45·9
5 – 9	107	8,895	12·0
10 – 14	49	8,355	5·9

Sixty-two of the children included in the survey were admitted to hospital as in-patients.

Falls were the commonest type of injury to children under 5, while cuts were the commonest among school children. Over a fifth of accidents to pre-school children were the result of swallowing substances, which included a range of medicines, contraceptive pills, cosmetics, detergents, paint, turpentine, paraffin, coins, screws, drawing pins, marbles and poppy seeds. There was a relatively low incidence of burns (5·6 per cent) and scalds (6·6 per cent). Nearly 5 per cent involved crushed fingers, usually in doors.

The writers pointed out that it is perhaps difficult for parents to realise the extent to which 2 or 3-year-olds can climb to obtain medicines, and suggest that copying adults was a causal factor in the case of the 3-year old boy who drank half a bottle of cherry brandy (he was admitted to hospital) and the 8-year-old, also admitted to hospital, who drank a bottle of port while his parents were asleep on a Sunday morning. They added the following comment:

'However conscientious parents may be and however effective any health education programme there is an element of unpredictability and an area where possible danger cannot be foreseen. Such was the case of a 3-month-old baby who was injured while held in his mother's arms. A gust of wind blew open the back door of the house causing a cupboard door by which the mother was standing to open violently, hitting the baby's head and fracturing its skull. Not only did this distress the parents but it was quite justifiably suspected by the Casualty Officer of being a case of baby battering. When the health visitor made enquiries, however, she found that it was an accident which could not possibly have been foreseen.'

If the back door, or the cupboard door, had been fitted with more effective latches this accident might not have happened. The incident may well illustrate poor engineering design rather than unpredictability.

From time to time fatal accidents occur in schools, involving roller-towels, trampolines, glass doors or even television trolleys, but such occurrences are fortunately rare.

In 1965 the Department of Education and Science, in conjunction with chief education officers, principal school medical officers and head teachers investigated all the accidents in maintained schools in ten local education authorities in England and Wales that caused fractured bones or an absence from school for half a day or longer. The results were published in *Health of the school child 1966–68* (see references). The child population included in the survey was approximately 834,000, or just over 11 per cent of the total maintained school population in 1965. During the year 4,058 children (2,586 boys and 1,472 girls) sustained accidents as defined above; 9 per cent of the children involved were admitted to hospital as in-patients.

The largest group of accidents was made up of those which happened in playgrounds, with playing fields the next most common location. Accidents in gymnasia comprised the third largest group, and those in classrooms the fourth. There were few accidents in home economics or handicraft rooms, laboratories or swimming baths, but rather more in cloakrooms, in corridors, and on steps.

More children were injured during physical education than during other teaching activities; the accident rates during physical education were considerably higher among older boys and girls, and higher among boys than girls.

No deaths occurred in the schools of the ten local education authorities concerned during 1965.

The commonest injuries were broken bones (40 per cent), followed by cuts and abrasions (32 per cent), dislocations and severe sprains (15 per cent), concussion and internal head injuries (5 per cent). There were very few serious burns and scalds. The variations between the areas covered by the survey were very marked, ranging from an incidence of 245·7 per 100,000 pupils to 790·0 accidents per 100,000 pupils. It is difficult to believe that so great a range is solely attributable to differences in material provision. It is tempting to speculate that it may have been due to differences in community awareness and to socio-economic factors, and that there may be a connection between these factors and the attitudes of people towards safety and health education.

If the figures obtained in this survey are extrapolated to cover all maintained schools in England and Wales they suggest that in 1965 about 35,000 children were injured in school, and that about 3,000 of them were admitted to hospital.

The report of this survey ends thus:

'Supervising active, lively children, especially in playgrounds, playing fields and gymnasia is onerous at all times, and it is impossible to prevent accidents ever occurring. School doctors should however, in collaboration with the teachers, study the circumstances under which injuries occur to see if accident prevention measures could be strengthened further.'

The following quotations from introductory sections to Department of Education and Science Safety Series No 4, No 3, and No 2 are relevant:

First: No. 4—*Safety in physical education*
'Physical education includes many activities which offer a challenge to the child's initiative, determination and courage. In some there is an element of danger, while others, although safe in themselves, are given a spice of adventure by being carried out under hazardous conditions. The personal risk involved in competitive games and in many outdoor pursuits is no doubt one reason for their wide appeal. Safety precautions cannot remove all risks, but should eliminate unnecessary dangers.

'The prevention of accidents largely depends on the skill, knowledge and example of the teacher, but he will remember always the need to develop a sense of responsibility among his pupils and an understanding of the importance of the part they play in ensuring their own safety, and that of their fellows. He will be aware of their ages and stage of training, and of their handicaps where they exist. Skilled movement, care and sensible use of the body, health and hygiene, how to keep the body fit for everyday living, are all aspects of education and safety towards which the physical education teacher will endeavour to develop positive attitudes.

'. . . If, in spite of everything, an accident should happen the teacher must know exactly what to do, and be able to recognise a situation in which medical help is necessary . . .'

Secondly: No. 3 *Safety in practical departments.*
'Teachers of all crafts are not only concerned with preventing accidents but also with safety education as an essential part of their work. There are more crippling and fatal accidents in the home than anywhere else, and a particularly disturbing feature of industrial accidents is the number which occur to young people under the age of eighteen, often in the early weeks of first employment. Not only, therefore, must home economics, art and craft rooms and workshops be planned and equipped with safety principles in mind, allowing effective supervision, easy access to all sections of the working area and avoiding over-crowding, but pupils should be encouraged to develop confidence, mature assessment of potential danger, and a sense of responsibility for themselves and others.

'In every department there are certain safety rules which must be understood and observed . . .'

Thirdly: No. 2 *Safety in science laboratories*

'The purpose of paying attention to safety precautions is to foster proper and lasting attitudes of mind to safety and to increase the confidence of all who work in laboratories. It is the duty of those who design laboratories to do so with safe working in mind. Teachers and laboratory staff should attend to regular maintenance, and staff and pupils be alert to potential hazards so that they may be avoided. However, while known hazards can be guarded against there is always an element of unforeseen danger which calls for thoughtful and deliberate attitudes to laboratory work and the setting of good examples by teachers.'

The toll of accidents on the roads has aroused widespread public concern for at least two generations. The results of education, research into the causes of accidents and into ways of changing the environment (including both the design of roads and the design of vehicles) and legislation have combined to produce, at least in England and Wales, an almost static situation in the face of increasing road traffic.

The young pass through several recognisable phases in relation to road accidents. Pedestrians are most prone to road accidents when they are six, cyclists when they are 13, motor-cyclists when they are 17, and drivers between the ages of 20 and 25.

At first they are pedestrians only, and as we have seen, about 200 children under 5 die every year in England and Wales on the roads. Such tragedies are a consequence of failure of adult surveillance. The children are at hazard in an environment with which they cannot cope. A Transport and Road Research Laboratory (Department of the Environment) report of 1969, *Children and road safety: a survey amongst mothers*, points out that although mothers appear to accept that parents have the main responsibility for teaching children road safety, unaccompanied children continue to be killed on the roads. There was a marked discrepancy between what mothers thought and said about their children's safety on the road and what they did about it.

From the ages of 5 to 16 (phase two) children have to learn to use the roads safely as pedestrians and often as cyclists. And they are clearly in danger when the skills they have acquired are inadequate to meet unexpected and unfamiliar dangers. Disobedience, aggression, ignorance and temporary changes in the child's behaviour all contribute to a high-risk situation. One-third of all deaths to boys and girls between the ages of 5 and 15 are a consequence of traffic accidents. This does not imply criticism of teachers, or of others who help in the work of schools to promote road safety. Serious as the child casualty figures are, they would be much worse but for the devoted attention which teachers, with the skilled help of the police, give to prevention.

The third phase is that of beginning to drive, and it is widely known that young drivers, whose assurance often exceeds their judgement, patience and experience, are especially liable to accidents. This poses a problem which is almost entirely educational: the need for training in road sense—which begins early in life—inculcating driving skills, and encouraging sensible attitudes to driving behaviour, combining skill and acceptance of responsibility.

These points about accidents to children are summed up in the following quotations from a recent Swedish report (see references).

'The essential facts are simple: the infant's total dependence on supervision and protection, the toddler's dangerous and inexperienced activities, and the continuing discrepancy between the risks and awareness and respect for the risks in the growing child and adolescent all indicate that the basic principles of individual accident prevention must rest on constant supervision of the infant and training from early childhood onwards, to make the growing child successively more and more capable of assessing the risks and protecting himself by his own knowledge and experience . . .'

and

'As evidenced by all survey studies, the vast majority of childhood accidents result in minor injuries which might be preventable but only by heavily interfering with the child's normal behaviour and development. This is far from desirable. These minor injuries have in themselves an educational effect not only on the victims but also for their siblings, playmates etc, and for the parents giving everybody concerned a useful lesson hopefully increasing awareness of risks and safeguards.'

There remains the question of accident proneness, the notion of which is widely accepted by laymen and by insurance companies, whose statistics indicate a relationship between types of occupation and frequency of accidents to or caused by car drivers. A recent survey in Boston, Massachusetts showed that the use of seat-belts in cars is related to other preventative behaviour such as medical and dental check-ups, non-smoking, exercising and other good health habits.

The report *From birth to seven* by the National Children's Bureau (see references) quotes as an example of an 'obviously accident prone' child a boy who had burned his hand on a poker at 18 months; fallen off a donkey at 3, fracturing his collar bone; fallen into the water closet at 4, lacerating his scalp; and caught his arm in a washing machine a few months later.

Some authorities are reluctant to accept the concept of accident-proneness because it may lead to a fatalistic view of accidents. Klein, for example (see references), claims that the child who has frequent accidents is one who gets involved in environmental hazards more readily than other children, and argues that it makes little sense to concern ourselves with the accident-prone child but that it does make good sense to concern ourselves with the accident-inducing environment.

There appears to be little statistical evidence to decide the question, at least among children, but it is unwise to perpetuate the view that accident-prone behaviour is caused by deeply rooted psychological conflict, or by physical clumsiness, or by one of a variety of disorders of the central nervous system. It is more probable that the child whose motor skills have out-stripped his judgement is more frequently involved in accidents. But among adults obstinacy, absent-mindedness, poor eyesight, impaired hearing or sense of smell, dizziness or lack of physical co-ordination contribute to accidents. And road accidents sometimes occur when aggression is neither understood nor controlled. It may be that early recognition of the signs of tension, anger and hurt pride in children and young people, followed by methods of relieving them, is an important contribution to safety available to perceptive teachers and to parents.

When accidents happen, for whatever reason, it is vitally important that all teachers (and, as they grow older, all boys and girls), should know what to do. A knowledge of elementary first aid may make the difference between life and death. Simple ideas of first aid should be within the grasp of every boy and girl of secondary school age. But in considering what to include in a first aid course it is necessary to ask if there is a risk of inadequate first aid doing more harm than good. Children should not be trained to undertake responsibilities in advance of their years. They must realise that first aid has two main aims:

1. to recognise whether a particular injury needs more than simple attention,
2. to render such immediate help as will prevent aggravation of an injury or deterioration in the state of an injured person.

In both there are limits, which must be recognised, beyond which elementary first aid cannot go. The basic minimum for all teachers and older secondary pupils is summarised in the British Red Cross Society's leaflet *First aid at the roadside* under the headings Breathing Stopped; Bleeding; Unconsciousness; Fractures and General Care.

School is not the only place in which boys and girls can learn first aid. Many voluntary organisations offer instruction.

Life-saving from drowning is an important form of first aid. As many boys and girls as possible should be instructed in rescue and resuscitation, which have for years been practised with success by many schools. Here, too, faulty technique can be dangerous. If life-saving is taught it must be taught correctly and only when the essential proficiency in swimming has been reached.

The discussion of accident prevention (or minimisation) or safety education is confused by two distinct but not conflicting aims. The first is to protect children. It is obviously highly desirable that they shall survive to learn how to protect themselves. The second is to educate boys and girls so that they may cope with a hazardous environment and, in the long term, use their intelligence and ingenuity when they are grown up to make accidents less common than today, both by improving the environment (better design) and by collective agreement (legislation). These aims in a sense underlie all parts of health education.

When children are very young protection consists essentially in removing from their environment hazards which they cannot cope with. The responsibility rests with parents or guardians. But a stage is soon reached when children must begin to be trained in safety before they can fully understand the danger. For example, a child must be trained how to use mains electrical apparatus safely before he can possibly understand the properties of alternating currents at high voltages. This too is a responsibility of the home, which is gradually shared with the school. This phase merges into a period of growing understanding and acquisition of skills which demand, as time goes on, expert teaching which may be incidental to the work of teachers of, for example, science, home economics and physical education; or may be a responsibility shared by the class teacher and visiting experts, such as the police, when ideas of road safety are developed. This educational process is continuous and should lead to an increase in skill and in confidence. Such education (which is given not only by the home and school but also by youth organisations and, in the later stages, institutions of further education and work-places of many kinds) continues side by side with efforts to satisfy the first aim—to protect children and young people. But discretion and judgement have to be used to decide the appropriate degree of protection at any stage because no human activity is risk free. Throughout this aspect of preparation for living, judgement is also demanded of teachers and others to assess what levels of comprehension and skill can be achieved by each individual pupil.

The knowledge required in this, as in all other aspects of health education, is drawn from many subject areas. At the secondary stage physics teachers in particular have an important contribution to offer, while mathematicians can clarify the notion of risk and discuss with their pupils what probabilities of accidents of various kinds are widely regarded as acceptable, and why. A young man or woman who understands enough dynamics to realise the inevitable dissipation of energy when a large mass is suddenly brought to rest, to appreciate the significance of the relation between kinetic energy and velocity, the forces required to move a body in a curve, and the differences between rolling and sliding friction may drive with intelligence and understand the argument for wearing seat belts. A high proportion of accidents in the home, in the hills and on water are partly caused by ignorance of elementary science. The reader will find it instructive to construct a table showing the principles of physics neglected in such accidents as falling down the stairs, slipping on a mat on a polished floor, electrocution from an electrical appliance misused in a bathroom, capsizing a boat, getting lost in mist, dying from exposure in mountainous country, and many others. He may also like to consider the extent to which science, especially chemistry, can contribute to an understanding of the causes of many accidents—including scalding—due to combustion or to changes of physical state, so that casualties from fire and heat may be lessened. But, as in other areas of health education, knowledge and skill are not enough.

References

Statistical review of England and Wales, 1971, Registrar General (Office of Population Censuses and Surveys), HMSO, 1971.

'Table 8—Death by cause at ages under 15' in *The health of the school child 1971–72*, DES, HMSO, 1974.

'Home accidents to children under 15 years: Survey of 910 Cases', in *British medical journal*, vol. 3 pp 103–106, R Murdock and J Eva, BMA, 1974.

'Accidents at school', Ch. XI in *The health of the school child 1966–68*, DES, HMSO, 1969.

Safety Series

No. 1 *Safety in outdoor pursuits*, DES, HMSO, 1977 New Ed.

No. 2 *Safety in science laboratories*, DES, HMSO, 1976 New Ed.

No. 3 *Safety in practical departments*, DES, HMSO, 1973.

No. 4 *Safety in physical education*, DES, HMSO, 1975 Revised.

No. 6 *Safety at school: general advice*, DES, HMSO, 1977.

Prevention of childhood accidents in Sweden, T Ehrenpreis MD, Swedish Inst. for the Prevention of Accidents, 1972.

Who is to blame for childhood injuries? (Transactions of National Safety Congress, 1971), Klein.

From birth to seven, National Children's Bureau, Longman, 1972.

Accident proneness, L Shaw and H S Sichel, Pergamon, 1971.

Further reading

Education for hazards: the involvement of the doctor as a teacher (Report of symposium, Brighton, April, 1970), Royal College of Surgeons, Medical Commission on Accident Prevention.

'Home Accidents and Health Education' in *Health education journal* vol. 33, Nos. 2 and 3, HEC Medical Research Division, Health Education Council, 1974.

9

DENTAL HEALTH

Past surveys have shown that there was less decay in children's teeth during the war and the period of food rationing which followed it than there is today. From about 1950 the health of children's teeth in general deteriorated, but the most recent quinquennial survey conducted in 1973 by selected authorities for the Department of Education and Science (see references) shows that among 5-year-olds the gradual improvement which had been noticed since 1958 has continued and that the general dental condition in the young is now better than at any time since 1948. Completely sound teeth were found in 27·8 per cent of children in this group, while the average number of decayed, missing or filled teeth per child was 3·6. The comparable figures for 1958 were 12·8 per cent and 5·7 respectively. But only a very minor improvement was recorded in the 12-year-old group and the prevalence of dental caries among them remains high. Inflammation of the gums was discernible in more than half of the children by the age of 7. Gingivitis in children is often temporary and may be associated with the shedding or eruption of teeth. Among 12–14 year olds only 3 per cent had severe inflammation of the gums.

In recent years the average sugar consumption per head has not changed significantly but the proportion in the form of glucose included in processed foods has almost doubled since 1955. This may be a contributory factor in the reduction of dental caries in the 5-year-olds but the main reason for the decline is most probably more effective education of many mothers of young children. Considerable success has been achieved in teaching mothers the dangers of giving children undiluted fortified vitamin syrups especially in reservoir feeders so that the gross destruction, particularly of the upper front deciduous teeth, so common a few years ago is now seldom seen.

As the figures for the 12-year-olds indicate, this improvement does not appear to be maintained once the children are at school and away from continuous parental supervision. There is no doubt that the consumption of sweet sticky foods between meals is dentally most damaging. While recognising that in some cases school tuck shops usefully contribute to school life, efforts should be made to limit sales to foods such as nuts, crisps and fruit.

Prevention must be preferable to cure. Fluoridation of the public water supply at a concentration of one part per million is now widely held to be beyond reasonable doubt both safe and effective in reducing the onset of dental caries and this measure is being progressively introduced by a number of authorities. But its lack of universal adoption, for reasons to be discussed later, has prompted interest in other preventive measures. Experiments have been made into the effectiveness of applying fluoride in solution or as a gel to the surface of the teeth, and in using a mouth rinse containing fluoride in schools. More recently a plastic coating has been developed which can be used to seal the susceptible fissures in teeth. So far the long-term effects of these methods are inconclusive, while their cost, particularly in professional time, limits their suitability for widespread adoption.

The four rules of good dental health that have for long been taught are:
1. to eat nourishing meals, but nothing sweet or sticky between meals;
2. to brush the teeth and gums after breakfast and always last thing at night;
3. to finish meals with raw fruit or vegetables or rinse the mouth with water;
4. to visit the dentist regularly.

Modern dental health training concentrates on plaque control and on encouraging children to visit the dentist. Plaque is a deposit of bacteria, mucin, enzymes and food debris which forms on the teeth and is invisible in the early stages. It is the causative agent in dental caries, gingivitis, and, later in life, periodontal disease, in the long term the most serious disease as it is not easily detected until it causes gross and often irreparable damage. Plaque may be made visible by staining with so-called 'disclosing' agents which are available from pharmacists, so that children may see it and then remove it by effective brushing. Effective brushing invariably requires movement from the gums to the teeth and removal of all stained plaque. Once the technique has been mastered and established as a habit all that need be done is to check the possible growth of new plaque by applying a disclosing agent at intervals of several months. This will at least add greatly to the efficiency of teeth cleaning.

Dental caries is mainly a disease of childhood and adolescence. Periodontal disease, which attacks the tissues which support the teeth so that they eventually fall out, is an affliction of middle age. Both are caused by bacteriological action—in caries by attacking the teeth, in periodontal disease by attacking the gums. Bacteria, suspended in the plaque, ferment sugar from food and release acids close to the surface of the teeth. The bacteria are deprived of fermentable sugars by reducing the input of sugar, especially between meals when the production of saliva, which helps to remove food particles adhering to teeth, is low, and by the systematic mechanical (tooth brushing) removal of plaque. Plaque is also the removable cause of periodontal disease.

Pierre Fauchard, an eminent French dentist, remarked in 1746:

'The most common cause of the loss of teeth is the negligence of those people who do not clean their teeth when they might, and that they fail to perceive the lodgement of the foreign substance which produces disease on the gums.'

Dental health is increasingly being chosen as a topic for project work, especially in primary schools, but children need to be reminded repeatedly to care for their teeth. They can also be helped to realise the value of dental inspection and treatment; the purpose of both should be explained to them. Much useful dental educational material, including films, film strips, books and charts, is available to teachers from several sources.

The long drawn out controversy about the artificial fluoridation of drinking water as an effective way of reducing the onset of dental caries (not periodontal disease) has been referred to earlier. By August 1973 in England 98 authorities had declared themselves in favour, 82 against, five had not decided, and two believed that the natural fluoride content of their water supply was adequate. The decision, however, rested with the Water Boards, who would not act unless all the authorities served by them agreed—so the number of authorities in which action had been taken was far fewer than 98. The decision now rests with the area health authorities who may request regional water authorities to make the necessary arrangements.

Reduced to essentials the facts are as follows: fluorine is a very active element, found in compounds such as fluorspar (calcium fluoride), apatite (mixed calcium phosphate and fluoride) and cryolite (a compound of sodium, aluminium and fluorine). These naturally occurring substances are very plentiful in some parts of the world and, although they are not very soluble, water which percolates through rocks containing them takes up a low concentration of fluoride ions. In the United Kingdom the concentration of fluoride in drinking water is usually about $0 \cdot 1$ of a part per million but in a few areas the proportion is much higher. Fluoride is also contained in food, especially in some kinds of seafish, and it is absorbed from the soil by plants of the tea family. In the United States the daily intake from food has been estimated as being between $0 \cdot 2$ and $0 \cdot 8$ milligrams, but in England and Wales the range is higher, with an estimated maximum of $1 \cdot 8$ milligrams, because of the higher average consumption of tea.

The suggestion that a connection existed between fluoride in the diet and good dental health was first made in the 1890's. By 1901 stained teeth had been observed (this staining is nowadays referred to as mottling, which may be a symptom of dental fluorosis) at Colorado Springs (United States) where the concentration of fluoride ions in the water is relatively high ($2 \cdot 5$ parts per million). Mottling is now known to occur in some individuals whatever the concentration of fluoride, but it is generally more severe at higher concentrations. A series of studies in the United States, England and elsewhere—especially the *21 City Study* by Tendley Dean in the United States, discussed in *WHO Monograph No 59* (see references)—have pointed to the conclusion that if everyone who lives in a temperate climate drank water with a concentration of one part per million of fluoride throughout childhood and adolescence the incidence of dental caries would be halved, mainly because small quantities of fluoride help the body to build a good enamel barrier on the teeth, while mottling would be insignificant. Naturally such studies, both retrospective and prospective, are complicated by several variables which the reader may care to list for himself. References to some of this research are given at the end of the chapter. There is no suggestion that lack of fluoride ions causes dental caries. The conclusion is that fluoride, in this small concentration, strengthens the defences.

The following data (from Professor D Jackson, University of Leeds) give one example of many similar statistics:

Table VII
Average cumulative number of teeth with caries per person

age	York	Hartlepool
5	4·09	1·49
15	8·95	4·96
15–19	11·60	6·00
20–24	14·10	7·80

The fluoride content of drinking water in York is in the range 0·15–0·25 parts per million: in Hartlepool the natural level is about 1·90 parts per million.

There are other relevant facts. If the fluoride intake reaches 8 milligrams a day mottling of the teeth may cause significant disfigurement. People who have ingested 20–80 milligrams a day for 20 years have suffered from skeletal fluorisos, a crippling disease. Fatal doses are in the range 2·5–5·0 grams. There is an area of uncertainty about the extent, if any, to which prolonged periods of regular low doses of fluoride may disturb normal metabolism: fluoride is a known enzyme inhibitor which can work at very low concentrations. The argument is therefore mainly about concentration and safe levels and whether an extra unavoidable daily dose from the water supply might put a few people at risk. The contribution of water with a concentration of one part per million to the daily intake of fluoride ions is one milligram in each litre. To put this in the simplest terms the water in a cup of tea adds about 0·2 milligram of fluoride to the diet at places where it is fluoridated to the level generally accepted as sufficient to halve the incidence of dental caries in children. This would increase the intake of fluoride from a cup of tea from about 0·3 milligram to 0·5 milligram. So, in order to be at the slightest risk from skeletal fluorisis, it would be necessary to drink at least 40 cups of tea a day for 20 years, whereas if fluoride were not added to the water 60 cups a day could safely be consumed. A fatal dose would need the rapid consumption of at least 5,000 cups of tea made from fluoridated water—rapid consumption would be essential because only a minute proportion of fluoride is absorbed by the body, in teeth and in bone.

The World Health Organisation Assembly 1969 passed a resolution recommending fluoridation as a desirable measure after careful scrutiny of the evidence from many countries. This measure is also supported by the Central Health Services Council, the Standing Dental and Medical Advisory Committees, the British Medical Association, the British Dental Association, the Royal Society of Health, and the Royal College of Physicians. A recent report (1976) of the Royal College of Physicians concludes: 'There is no evidence that the consumption of water containing approximately 1 milligram per litre of fluoride in a temperate climate is associated with any harmful effect, irrespective of the hardness of the water'. Older boys and girls may find this unfinished story a useful and interesting example of interpretation of data and of decision making.

References

Children's dental health in England and Wales, Office of Population Censuses and Surveys, HMSO, 1973.

Dental health education 1970 (Technical report series No. 449), WHO, 1970.

Fluorides and human health 1970 (Monograph No. 59), (P Adley and others), WHO, 1970.

Fluoridation studies in the United Kingdom and results achieved after 11 *years* (Reports on Public Health and Medical Subjects No. 122), DHSS/Scottish Office/Welsh Office/Ministry of Housing and Local Government, HMSO, 1969.

'Dental Caries: Prospects for Prevention' in *Science* vol. 173 No. 4003, H W Scherp, American Assn. for the advancement of Science, 1971.

'Royal College of Physicians and Fluoridation' in *British medical journal* vol. 1 pp 57–58, BMA, 1976.

Fluoride, teeth and health, Royal College of Physicians, Pitman Medical, 1976.

Further reading

'Dental Health and Disease', Ch. 22 in *Man against disease*, A G Clegg and P C Clegg, Heinemann, 1973.

'Water Fluoridation: a Choice for the Community' in *Community health* vol. 6, Part 2, pp 75–83, J J Murray, John Wright and Sons Ltd., 1974.

10

THE MISUSE OF DRUGS

From time immemorial men and women have sought euphoria from drugs. Some drugs have been unacceptable in some cultures at some periods but have been openly used, although perhaps with restrictions, in other places and at other times. All drugs are potentially dangerous. The misuse of drugs, especially among the younger age groups, occurs nowadays to a greater or less extent in all technologically advanced countries. Public concern has led to the formation of a number of investigating committees and voluntary societies, to the holding of international conferences, and to the production of a mass of research papers and of teaching material of various kinds aimed at both teachers and pupils.

The Department of Health and Social Security (then the Ministry of Health) set up a Committee on the Safety of Drugs in 1964. This body defined a drug as

'any substance or mixture of substances destined for administration to man to use in the diagnosis, treatment, investigation or prevention of disease or for the modification of physiological functions'

This definition excludes cannabis, tobacco and alcoholic drinks. It has long been recognised that although a drug may be of value in treating a specific condition it could have undesirable and even dangerous effects on other parts of the body. Thalidomide drew public attention to the side effects of drugs in an unforgettable way, so a voluntary system for licensing new drugs was started in 1964—now changed to statutory licensing under the Safety of Medicines Committee. One reason for the great increase in the number of drugs is the search for precision in treatment with fewer side effects. Adverse reactions, unforeseen when a drug is introduced, can sometimes be identified only after extensive use.

The range of drugs available and the number prescribed have both increased very markedly since the 1939–45 war. In a recent research project (Durrell and Cartwright 1972—see references) the medicine-taking habits of a sample of the population were investigated. No less than 80 per cent of the adults in the sample had taken some medicine in the two weeks before they were interviewed, 55 per cent of them in the previous 24 hours. Among children, 55 per cent had been given medicine in the preceding two weeks. 20 per cent of the adults had taken four or five medicines. Analgesics (pain killers) were most frequently used, while 10 per cent had taken some form of psychotropic drug.

An increasing number of drugs is available for the treatment of the mentally ill and such drugs are also used to maintain everyday living by many anxious and disturbed people. As long ago as 1968 general practitioners issued, under the National Health Service, no less than 21 million prescriptions for hypnotics and sedatives a year, 16 million further prescriptions for tranquillizers, and five million for antidepressants, making in all 42 million prescriptions out of a total of 225 million for all drugs in the year—a change from the tons of bromide consumed before the war for similar reasons. Some of these drugs were almost certainly misused, and the process continues, giving rise to the non-therapeutic use of drugs. In this sense the word 'drugs' means substances which act on a person's central nervous system to produce changes in sensations, mood and perception. Such drugs need not have any recognised medical value, but the changes they induce are usually, at least in the early stages of use, pleasurable. This definition of drugs covers narcotics, stimulants, sedatives and hallucinogens, and includes cannabis alcohol and tobacco.

The concepts of dependence, escalation and tolerance are associated with drugs. Together they constitute the reasons why the use of some drugs, particularly those most liable to misuse, is subject to some form of control throughout the Western world.

Dependence has been defined in various ways. The most recent formal definition in World Health Organisation Technical Report Series No 407, 1969, is:

'A state, psychic and sometimes also physical, resulting from the interaction between a living organism and a drug, characterised by behavioural and other responses that always include a compulsion to take the drug on a continuous or periodic basis in order to experience its psychic effects, and sometimes to avoid the discomfort of its absence. Tolerance may or may not be present. A person may be dependent on more than one drug.'

This implies both physical and psychological dependence. There may be physiological changes produced in the body as a result of continued consumption of the drug, so that its withdrawal produces discomfort, and sometimes acute illness. There may also be a psychological craving for the drug which continues after the physical withdrawal symptoms have subsided.

Escalation expresses the idea that familiarisation with the so called 'soft' drugs predisposes the taker to the use of, and eventually to dependence on, 'hard' drugs. The words 'soft' and 'hard' have no precise meaning in this context—barbiturates when swallowed in therapeutically acceptable quantities may be regarded by some people as 'soft', but when injected are undoubtedly very 'hard'. Some observers regard the notion of escalation as no more than part of the mythology of the drug scene, but it is generally accepted that some people widen their repertoire and such 'poly drug users' often pose difficult problems. Most drug takers swallow or smoke drugs. A few eventually degenerate into 'fixing' by injection.

Tolerance means the development of resistance to the effects of a drug as use continues and the body adapts to it. So, if a drug is regularly consumed, the same dose produces less effect, or a larger dose is needed to produce the same effect. This phenomenon is well known to readers of detective stories in which morphia is used as a fatal poison.

A great deal of anxiety arises, especially in parents and others concerned for the welfare of young people, because of the association of these characteristics with the misuse of drugs, and they may not always realise that dependence—the main fear—varies from drug to drug and from person to person. One pill or one puff of cannabis is most unlikely to establish dependence and may even bring revulsion, just as one pint of beer does not inevitably lead to alcoholism. But there is, rightly, a general fear of getting 'hooked', a fear expressed by boys and girls as well as by their parents.

Dependence is a phenomenon which is not only associated with drugs. Psychological dependence can take many forms, some bizarre. Dependence on work is a psychological disturbance which affects some highly intelligent people with most uncomfortable consequences for those who have to live with them, while obsessive dependence on food in general, and substances like sugar in particular, is by no means uncommon.

Drugs which may be misused can be divided into five main classes.

1. Narcotics

This class includes opium (obtained from the opium poppy) with its derivatives morphine, heroin and codeine; and a group of synthetic substances of which the most common are methadone and pethidine. They are used medically to combat severe pain. Their immediate effect is to relieve pain, relax tension and give a pleasant feeling of euphoria. But the effect of a single dose soon wears off, and after a period of regular doses unpleasant withdrawal symptoms occur, so that the drugs can produce severe physical dependence.

The body soon develops tolerance to them, so that they are frequently injected to give a quicker and more satisfying reaction. Their use often therefore leads to the unpleasant and dangerous effects of non-sterile injections, such as abscesses and other infections such as septicaemia. It has been estimated that the death rate from heroin abuse is one in ten per year irrespective of the age of the victim. Death is usually the culmination of the effects of heroin on the body and of severe physical debility due to personal neglect. But the effects of heroin and the drugs associated with it often eventually compel the victim to seek help.

2. Stimulants

This class includes cocaine and the amphetamine group of drugs, commonly known as pep pills.

Cocaine, which occurs naturally as a constituent of the coca plant, was at one time used by people dependent on heroin to improve the initial effects and to reduce some of the withdrawal symptoms. It was also used from time to time in the last century and earlier in this century in some literary circles. At present its use is insignificant but may again become fashionable.

The amphetamines have been prescribed as anti-depressants, and as slimming pills because they suppress appetite. They temporarily ward off fatigue, and cause people to feel elated and able, in their own estimation, to talk and behave brilliantly: brilliance which may appear to others as truculence and aggression. Tolerance is common so that very large doses can eventually be taken, which may induce hallucinations and delusions of persecution, known as 'the horrors', with an aftermath of extreme fatigue and mental depression. The World Health Organisation classes amphetamines as drugs of psychological dependence. There are clearly very good reasons why amphetamines nowadays are very rarely prescribed.

3. Sedatives

The sedatives, such as barbiturates and methaqualone (mandrax) depress the action of the nervous system and so release inhibitions and lead to behaviour typical of a person who has drunk too much. Alcoholic drinks must also be classed as sedatives and a mixture of barbiturates with even moderate quantities of alcohol is very dangerous: according to dose such mixtures depress the brain's activity from sedation to coma and even death. Tolerance to barbiturates develops, with a tendency to increase the dose, and the drugs induce both physical and psychological dependence. Withdrawal symptoms following heavy dosage (misuse) can be very unpleasant and may well include epileptic fits, delirium, delusions of persecution and suicidal tendencies. It was estimated in 1970 that about 2 per cent of the population of England and Wales took barbiturates, accounting for 7 per cent of National Health Service prescriptions. Since then other sedatives and tranquillizers, believed neither to induce dependence nor to offer the prospect of successful suicide, have been prescribed to an increasing extent as safer substitutes for barbiturates.

Barbiturates are normally obtained as capsules or tablets which are swallowed, but some very disturbed drug abusers are known to mix them with water and inject them intravenously. This is a very dangerous practice as it may damage blood vessels and so cause chronic skin ulceration or even gangrene. Sometimes such an injection results in sudden death.

4. Hallucinogens

LSD (d-lysergic acid diethylamide) is the best known among a group of synthetic hallucinogens. A few doctors believe that it has value in the treatment of psychiatric disorder, but it is almost invariably illicitly manufactured and supplied. In many ways it is the most dangerous of the drugs subject to abuse. LSD is relatively easy to produce in commercial quantities, given some laboratory facilities and the necessary skill. The purity and strength of illicitly manufactured LSD is variable, which may lead to over-dosage, especially as the 'normal' dose is minute, ranging between 100 microgrammes and 1 milligram. The most dangerous factor, probably, is the variation in response from individual to individual and, in a given individual, from time to time, to the drug. Even with a mature personality a 'bad trip' can occur if the mood and environment are unfavourable. Hallucinogens, besides altering perception, impair judgement and sometimes give rise to fanciful ideas of physical capability which can lead to attempts at irrational feats that may cause severe injury or death to the drug taker or to others. The horror of a 'bad trip' can be psychologically damaging, and with LSD in particular a 'flash back' or 'repeat trip' can occur without warning weeks or even months after the drug was taken. Cases of prolonged psychotic illness have been reported following a single dose of LSD.

Cannabis can be included among the hallucinatory drugs although it also possesses some of the characteristics of the sedatives. It can be produced from the dried flowering tops of the Indian hemp plant (*cannabis sativa*) when it is called marihuana, or extracted from the plant as a resin known as hashish. Each form is usually smoked, mixed with tobacco, in a cigarette known as a 'reefer' or 'joint'. The smoking of cannabis appears to be the commonest initial form of experimenting with drugs by young people, who believe, or say that they believe, that cannabis, unlike alcohol and tobacco, is a safe drug.

Cannabis is no longer used in Western medicine. It is a complex substance including a psychically active chemical (tetrahydrocannabinol —THC) which is soluble in fat so that it and its metabolites persist in the body. In contrast to alcohol (which is metabolised rapidly and is therefore short term in its effects) the active principle of cannabis is only slowly excreted, and may accumulate in the body if regularly used.

The effects of cannabis depend on the circumstances in which it is taken and, as with other drugs, vary from person to person. It is said to induce a greater awareness of self and of the members of the group in which it is smoked, and a finer perception of colours and of music, leading to a state of sleepy stupor described as being 'stoned'. So although cannabis in some ways resembles LSD, its effect (unlike that of LSD) passes over into a sedative action which may be called intoxication.

The extent to which cannabis produces dependence—even the question whether it produces dependence or not—is still being debated, just as it was over 70 years ago by the witnesses before the Indian Hemp Commission.

The important practical question is whether it is harmful. The legal control of cannabis, exercised in many parts of the world, is an expression of the uncertainty which surrounds its long-term effects. No drug has been the object of so much research—pharmacological and social—in the past two decades. Among the most recent published statements are *Marihuana: a signal of misunderstanding* (1972) from the United States; *Cannabis: a report of the Commission of Inquiry into the non-medical use of drugs* (1972) from Canada, and a substantial section of *Drug trafficking and drug abuse* (1971) from Australia (see references). It is possible to tear quotations from their context in these and other writings to support almost any point of view. All that can be said with confidence is that the uncertainty persists. But there have been occasional reports of cannabis psychosis and it has recently been suggested that cerebral changes have followed prolonged heavy use. There is little doubt that regular users over several years in the Middle East and India cease to be productive members of the community, but this may be due to extremes of poverty, disease and inertia. There is accumulating evidence that regular heavy use by young people may lead to apathy and social deterioration. It certainly remains to be proved that cannabis cannot damage the brain or induce cancers. There is no evidence that cannabis, by its nature, induces escalation to other drugs: but it is highly probable that enjoyment of the first drug, often cannabis, may encourage experiments with others.

5. Glues and Solvents

Glues and solvents are sometimes 'sniffed' because they contain volatile substances such as amyl alcohol (used in modelling glues), tetrachlorethylene (commonly used in cleaning fluids) and volatile anaesthetics such as trichlorethylene and ether. These depress the nervous system. The misuse of household chemicals in this way is a strange aberration, not uncommon in North America and not unknown in the United Kingdom, and occurs usually in children or young adolescents. The danger in breathing even small quantities of these or other household fluids is not in dispute and it can cause unconsciousness and perhaps death. Long-term 'sniffing' damages the liver. kidneys and nervous system.

The extent of drug misuse, especially among young people (some of whom may still be at school) is impossible to judge because the practice, being illegal, is not widely admitted. The only figures available are for registered opiate addicts who are maintained by having their drug needs prescribed legally to keep them from progressive degradation. From 1945 to 1960 there were between 400–500 registered narcotic addicts in England and Wales, mostly middle aged or elderly people, many of whom were members of professions which had access to drugs. From 1960 until 1969 the figures rose because of an increase in addiction among the 17–25 year age group. In 1968 a programme was started to combat this growth of dependence on narcotics among young people. Treatment Units were established and new regulations for the registration of opiate addicts were brought into force. By 1970 the total number registered was about 1,500, and since then the figure appears to have stabilised. There was a marked decline in the number of people under 20 registered in the period 1969–73, as shown in Table VII below:

Table VII
Number of registered narcotics addicts in the ages 14, 15, 16, 17, 18, 19

| | | | 1969–1972 age | | | | |
	14	15	16	17	18	19	Total
1969	0	0	24	83	218	312	637
1970	0	1	9	49	117	229	405
1971	0	0	10	45	114	169	338
1972	1	1	7	27	85	158	279

This shows that the probability of a boy or girl at school becoming dependent on a narcotic is remote.

The only other relevant data are the number of prosecutions for drug offences and the quantities of drugs impounded by the police. Both sets of data show marked and continuing increases in the past few years, which may in part be because police drug squads have become more experienced.

Several small scale enquiries designed to estimate the extent of drug misuse among school boys and girls and among students have recently been made, using the technique of questionnaire and interview applied to samples. Such investigations, especially among school children, are extremely difficult and some may question their desirability. Boys and girls may choose not to be frank about practices which are illegal and which are disapproved of by the great majority of adults. But such enquiries, combined with the knowledge acquired by teachers, parents, social workers and the police make it clear that school children often have access to drugs. The position in 1975 appeared to indicate that many boys and girls have the opportunity to experiment with drugs, which they ignore or soon abandon; that some join a minority who are attracted especially to cannabis or LSD; and that very few indeed step into dependence on heroin or its associates. There is a wide variation from area to area in the extent of such experimenting, which depends, presumably at least in part, on the availability of supplies. There are also changes from year to year. Local outbreaks occur, which, like outbreaks of other contagious diseases, grow and then gradually die away. There is also at least the possibility of changes in fashion (some drugs may be 'in') and there was an indication a few years ago that amphetamines, which are now much more difficult to obtain, were popular among boys and girls determined on a lively weekend while cannabis, and occasionally LSD, had more appeal to students. There is evidence which indicates that the great majority of boys and girls are well aware both of the differences between the effects of different drugs and of the dangers of dependence, and have pity or contempt for those who are 'hooked': but at the same time are willing to experiment—often as part of a group activity—in practices which they may believe offer little risk.

Attempts to control drug abuse
The nineteenth report of WHO Expert Committee on Drug Dependence (1973) includes an interesting account of the methods and difficulties of epidemiological work on the misuse of drugs.

Legislation may be directed at the traders by imposing controls on the manufacture, import, distribution, prescription, price, or time of sale; or at the possessors or the consumers of a drug. Just as legislation seeks to control the use of alcohol and, in England and Wales, the sale of tobacco to children under the age of 16, so to a much stronger degree legislation is applied throughout the world to the control of drugs capable of misuse.

A number of Acts controlling the possession and sale of drugs were consolidated, and to some extent amended, in the Misuse of Drugs Act 1971, which came into force in 1973. This Act, like its predecessors, makes it an offence to possess, without authority, narcotics, cocaine, cannabis, amphetamines and LSD and other hallucinogens. Barbiturates are not controlled except that they may only be retailed by an authorised pharmacist on a prescription given by a medical practitioner.

The Act makes it possible for the Home Secretary to control new drugs and other substances by regulation without the need for new substantive legislation, and makes clear distinction between the offence of illegal possession and the offence of trafficking. The Act also made provision for the formation of an Advisory Council on the Misuse of Drugs, which is now established.

There is a great deal of co-operation to minimise the trade in illegal drugs. At an international level the World Health Organisation Expert Committee on Drug Dependence advises governments both directly, and indirectly by the issue of a series of authoritative reports. The police forces of England and Wales have drug squads responsible for the prevention of trafficking and for unlawful use. Members of these squads are concerned for the welfare of young people caught up in the drug scene, and co-operate with head teachers and others whose work brings them into contact with such boys and girls. Many local authorities have set up liaison committees, composed of members of statutory and voluntary bodies and others who work with young people, to monitor and, if necessary, to combat the threat of drug misuse.

Why drug abuse?
Many attempts have been made by doctors, teachers and sociologists in several countries to understand why some boys and girls misuse drugs. The simplest reason is that they enjoy, at least for a time, the physical and mental sensations induced by drugs. Like alcohol, drugs can be a means of boosting self-confidence in social situations; pep pills have the added attraction of keeping the party lively. Curiosity, very understandable in a period when inquiry and experiment are encouraged in many aspects of school life, is another motive. Drug taking may be associated with the behaviour of what appears a particularly attractive group of contemporaries, especially attractive if the group is in revolt against the conventions of adult society. For some young people there is a pleasure in secrecy—something secret and special to themselves—and in the added thrill of risk of discovery. Others enjoy ritual: cannabis smoking is often associated with group rituals (see, for example, *Marihuana: a signal of misunderstanding*). They may believe that cannabis makes the guitar sound more tuneful and the grass look greener—as well it may.

If these are the only factors which attract the adolescent into drug experimentation it is most likely that, in the words of Dr P Boyd (see references):

'. . . he will be one of the great majority of young people who draws back before he becomes the slave to his own adventure. Emotionally normal and mature individuals practically never become addicted, nor do adolescents who are making sound progress in their development towards maturity'.

Drugs, to such boys and girls, are but another hazard in the process of growing up. But if a boy or girl feels compelled to take drugs to bolster himself in the context of his development the risk changes profoundly. The pleasure and relief from anxiety obtained from drugs may lead to them being used in an attempt to solve problems, developing into a means of avoiding problems, so that drugs become the apparent escape route when problems are overwhelming. Drugs may then offer a means of destroying something within the self with which he cannot come to terms. At times this destruction becomes that of the whole person and reflects an ultimate despair which haunts some youngsters during adolescence but which seldom comes out into the open. Drug taking can then take on what Dr Boyd describes as the 'dimension of a chronic unconscious suicidal event', and the victim may then inject himself regularly with narcotics. The social and educational problem is to avoid such disasters, without exaggerating the consequences of occasional experiments or occasional folly. There is also a real danger that over-emphasis in teaching about drugs may arouse curiosity and a wish to experiment in young people who have not previously thought about such things.

The teacher's role in combating drug abuse
Teachers are advised not to rely on signs of drug abuse such as injection

marks or the characteristic smell of burning cannabis which are so easily recognised that few boys and girls would be so foolish as not to keep them hidden. More useful clues are changes of behaviour—especially behaviour which becomes uncharacteristic of the child—and a developing pattern of behaviour likely to interfere with his educational progress and social growth. In these circumstances teachers should seek medical advice. They should realise that the changes which have alerted them may be nothing to do with drugs, but may be signs of maladjustment. If maladjusted boys and girls are not treated there is an added risk of their experimenting and becoming dependent on drugs.

The teacher's role in dealing with drug misuse has a direct and an indirect aspect. The direct aspect is to strengthen relationships of trust and understanding with young people in what is still a highly charged area and to open up discussion. Exhortation, as in all other aspects of health education, is unlikely to be useful. It will help teachers if they are clear in their own minds on two points—first on the fact that the increasing variety of drugs available is the result of technical development which all boys and girls have to learn to live with and therefore need to understand; and secondly, on the nature of their own objectives in any teaching and discussion about drug misuse.

Teaching and discussion about drugs have a place in education at all stages of school life—not in the form of a terrifying film show or a lecture from a visiting expert as a reaction to a real or imagined crisis, but as a part of health education. From an early age children should know, and therefore must be taught by parents and by teachers, that pills and medicines must never be taken without their parents' knowledge, and then only the dose prescribed by the doctor. They should be taught never to sniff or taste any substances not recognised as food. At a later stage the ideas of dependence, escalation and tolerance can be discussed rationally, while the dangers of self-medication, even to the taking of vitamin pills, are pointed out.

As boys and girls grow up they should learn something of the ways in which laws are decided upon and about the extent of international agreement and co-operation over drug misuse—the law on drugs represents a consensus of opinion, revised from time to time to protect society. They will also come to appreciate that euphoria has been sought in various ways by successive generations—that in a given society some, but not all, euphoriants, are socially acceptable. But even socially acceptable drugs have long-term dangers and everyone has to decide for himself the extent to which he will use them, and the extent to which society requires him to limit their use for its protection. At a more advanced level, especially if they are embarking on a serious study of the humanities, children will learn that many talented artists, writers and musicians have claimed enhancement of vision and insight by drugs. But discussion with a skilled teacher will soon dispel the idea that mediocrity may be converted into genius by chemicals. And boys and girls, especially those most impatient with adult values and the 'consumer society' will readily appreciate that the trade in illegal drugs is a profitable racket organised by unscrupulous adults who prey on the young for gain, and realise that they are neither sensible nor consistent if they allow their impatience with adult values to lead them to be exploited by such means.

The indirect aspect of the teacher's work in the prevention of drug misuse—which he shares with parents and all others concerned for the welfare of growing boys and girls—is to create, so far as he is able, a climate which may at least make recourse to drugs less probable. It may be helpful, for example, in the school, as in the home, to give as much reassurance as possible in social situations. The belief of generations of teachers that they are right to encourage among their pupils constructive group activities which are not interfered with by adults may be reaffirmed.

Teachers will appreciate that many boys and girls need support in moments of uncertainty and self doubt. Probably the best support is an awareness of success. Every boy and girl, however unskilled or slow, needs to be seen by his peers to achieve something and needs praise for his or her achievement, however modest. They will also realise that stress may become overwhelming, through the culmination of difficulties at home, persistent unkindness or even the extreme pain of rejection. Unattainable academic goals, set by parents or by teachers, may create a sense of responsibility and of failure which can become intolerable. A great deal may be achieved, and undoubtedly is achieved, by teachers in the exercise of imagination and constructive sympathy in such circumstances. Nothing will be achieved by those who resort to exhortation especially if their pupils have good cause to believe that they know very little about drugs.

When pupils are found to be experimenting with drugs the responsibility to decide the wisest course of action rests with heads of schools. An incident of drug misuse should not provoke a witch hunt. There is a sensitive area of trust between adults and young people. Adult scrutiny, especially if surreptitious, brings a hostile reaction from young people. Parents are likely to be confused and distressed, and there may be acute conflict between parent and child. More objectivity can be expected from heads. There is much to be said for a cooling-off period, for keeping a sense of proportion, and for knowing when and where to seek expert help. Several local education authorities have established 'hot lines' between heads of schools and designated medical practitioners for use in such situations. It is most important that school children found to be experimenting with drugs should not be ostracised and thus forced into a position of being accepted only by a drug-orientated sub-culture. The police are especially concerned with the detection of the sources of drugs.

If there is evidence that members of a school are involved in drug taking the possibility that the source of their supplies may be some person in the neighbourhood, adult or juvenile, cannot be ignored. When heads are certain that drugs are being misused by members of their schools they have a duty to inform the police.

References

Amphetamines, barbiturates, LSD and cannabis—their use and misuse, DHSS, HMSO, 1970.
Reports on Public Health No. 124
Technical Report Series:
No. 273, WHO Expert Committee on Drug Dependence, WHO, 1964.
No. 407, WHO Expert Committee on Drug Dependence, WHO, 1969.
No. 460, WHO Expert Committee on Drug Dependence, WHO, 1970.
No. 526, WHO Expert Committee on Drug Dependence, WHO, 1973.
Drug trafficking and drug abuse, Australian Govt. Pub. Service, Australian Govt. Pub. Service, 1971.

Cannabis—a report of the Commission of Enquiry into the non-medical use of drugs, Canadian Government, Canadian Government, 1972.
Marihuana—a signal of misunderstanding (Report of the National Commission on Marihuana and Drug Abuse), United States Government, 1972.
'Heroin Addiction in Adolescence', in *Journal of psychosomatic medicine*, P. Boyd, 1970.
Medicine takers, prescribers and hoarders, K Dunnell and A Cartwright, Routledge and Kegan Paul, 1972.

Further reading

Where on drugs: a parents' handbook, B McAlhone (Ed.), ACE, 1970.
Drugs: the parents' dilemma (4th Ed.), A R K Mitchell, Priory Press, 1972.
Drug problems and their management, D Richter, Association for the Prevention of Addiction, 1970.
Connexions—out of your mind, P Newmark, Penguin, 1970.
Para. 3. 48 (background information) in *Biology of man*—Secondary Science 3, Nuffield Foundation, Longman, 1971.

'Nerves and Movement', Ch. 5 in *Advanced biology: study guide*, Nuffield Foundation, Longman, 1970.
'Drug Misuse" by Dr J Ward, Appendix to Curriculum Paper 14, *Health education in schools*, Scottish Education Department, HMSO, 1974.
Planning teaching about drugs, alcohol and cigarettes (Information/Education Series), Institute for the Study of Drug Dependence, 1974.
Education and drug dependence, Social Morality Council, Methuen Educational, 1975.

11

ALCOHOLIC DRINKS

Alcoholic drinks are by far the commonest drugs used by adults in many, but not all, parts of the world. The great majority recognise that such drinks can be misused and have accepted for generations legal controls on their use: a minority in England and Wales and elsewhere believe that their consumption cannot be justified in any circumstances.

Alcoholic drinks differ from the drugs discussed in the previous chapter in several respects. Knowledge of their properties has been gained over many centuries; their use is widespread and is often associated with happy social and family events; their production and distribution is a legal and reputable part of international industry and trade. Many adults, probably a majority in the Western world, believe that alcoholic drinks can be enjoyed in moderation in ways which cannot reasonably be described as irresponsible. Whatever opinion is held or whatever principle is maintained the fact is that alcoholic drinks are, and may be expected to continue to be, part of the social environment in which young people grow up and are yet another potential hazard to their health which they have to learn to live with.

Alcohol (ethanol) is not a drink. But beers and wines, made by fermentation, contain between 4 and 7 per cent and 10 and 20 per cent of ethanol respectively, while spirits, made by distillation, have an ethanol content in the range 40–55 per cent. Fermentation in the process of wine making ceases when the concentration reaches 15 per cent so some wines, such as sherry and port, are made stronger (fortified) by the addition of brandy. The rest is nearly all water. The compounds which sometimes defy analysis but give each drink its character are present in very small quantities, but the products of fermentation and distillation taste very different from solutions of pure ethanol.

All alcoholic drinks depress the activity of the higher centres of the brain so that inhibitions are lessened and social intercourse generally becomes easier. Increasing amounts progressively impair judgement, sometimes causing loss of temper or other forms of aggressive behaviour, and reduction of the ability to perform intricate physical movements resulting in clumsiness and slurring of speech. Further stages of intoxication cause the typical staggering gait of the drunkard and may lead to unconsciousness and death. It is impossible to be precise about the concentrations of alcohol in the blood which produce these various effects or about the rate at which alcohol is absorbed into the blood stream. In England and Wales a concentration of 80 milligrams of alcohol per 100 millilitres of blood is the limit above which it is illegal to drive a vehicle. At a level of about 550 milligrams per 100 millilitres, unconsciousness, or even death, may occur—a concentration which (depending on body weight) can be reached by drinking about 15 pints of beer or a bottle of whisky. Unconsciousness or death is not the invariable consequence of such heavy drinking, because tolerance slowly develops towards alcohol, as towards other drugs. Alcohol, unlike the active principle of cannabis, is rapidly eliminated from the body, but in some individuals stabilisation with a significant concentration of alcohol in the blood may be established after heavy drinking for some years. This can lead to physical defects such as gastritis and liver cirrhosis. Liver cirrhosis can develop rapidly when alcohol becomes a substitute for food because there is then too little an intake of vitamins and amino-acids.

Drunkenness and alcoholism
In considering the misuse of alcohol it is important to distinguish between drunkenness and alcoholism. Drunkenness is episodic, sometimes messy, humiliating, and hazardous, but soon recovered from. Milder states of intoxication than drunkenness are incompatible with effective work and add to the risks of accidents on the road and in the home.

Alcoholism, which most physicians and psychiatrists nowadays regard as a disease, is an extremely damaging state of dependence on alcohol. It is not an easy condition to define. The World Health Organisation regards alcoholics as

'those excessive drinkers whose dependence on alcohol has attained such a degree that it shows a noticeable mental disturbance of and interference with their bodily and mental health, their personal relationships and their smooth economic functioning, or who show the prodromal signs of such development. They therefore need treatment.'

Perhaps it is simpler to regard an alcoholic as someone whose drinking is completely out of hand. Some observers are prepared to accept, as a quantitative definition, that an alcoholic is a man or woman whose regular daily input of alcohol exceeds 150 millilitres, ie about two-thirds of a bottle of spirits. No matter what definition is adopted the victim is dependent on a drug to a degree which seriously disturbs his own life and the life of his family, so he needs treatment.

The approach of alcoholism is usually slow, gradual and insidious. Most alcoholics are middle aged but there is now a group of young alcoholics, disturbed young people who are sometimes also dependent on other drugs. Efforts to end dependence on barbiturates or other drugs can lead to dependence on alcohol—and vice versa.

A decline into alcoholism is often difficult to observe because the victim is at pains to disguise his condition and because his relatives and friends are often reluctant to admit that a problem exists. But most workers in this field accept that there are between 300,000 and 400,000 alcoholics in England and Wales. Over 10,000 are admitted each year to the 18 alcoholic treatment units or to psychiatric hospitals. There is no recognisable 'alcoholic personality' although some occupations are more heavily represented than others. There is no known biological reason why a small minority of drinkers is at such grave risk. International surveys show very marked national variations.

Some observers believe that different ethnic groups learn to drink in different ways and that further data, followed by further study of these differences, may point to ways of minimising the risk. There are many different drinking customs. In some countries drinking is a social activity confined largely to the club or pub, while in others, where wine has been plentiful for generations, alcoholic drink is more likely to be regarded as an essential companion to food. All countries in which alcoholic drinks are available have a small minority of solitary drinkers who turn to alcohol to anaesthetize themselves.

There has been a long history of legislation to control drinking in England and Wales, especially during the nineteenth century, when repeated efforts were made to reduce widespread drunkenness. Essentially legislation consisted in taxation, the control of sales, and punishment for drunkenness—principles which continue to this day—measures very strongly supported by generations of workers in the temperance movement. Convictions for drunkenness in England were about 200,000 a year at the beginning of this century. Lloyd George, perhaps mindful of the loss of production in munitions factories caused by drunkenness, regarded drink as a greater foe than Germany, so that in 1915 a Liquor Traffic Control Board was established which imposed a drastic reduction in licensing hours, restrictions on the supply of liquor, and even heavier taxation. Whatever the causes there was a very marked fall in drunkenness from the First World War until the 1950's. But the consumption of alcohol has risen sharply in the last decade, and in particular, wine, which used to be regarded as elitist, is now drunk more frequently than in any period since the 17th century. Vodka is gaining in popularity among young people, especially young women. Most important, there is an increasing suspicion that boys and girls of school age, who are not permitted to drink in public, are in fact experimenting and frequently acting illegally in so doing, to an extent which would not have been tolerated a few years ago. Observation in 1975 showed no certainty of a trend in adolescent behaviour which might lead to an alarming situation, but teachers, parents and others will wish to be alerted to the possibility. Generalisations about the behaviour of young people are invariably unwise, and what is now feared by some observers may well turn out to be a passing fashion embraced by a minority. All that can be stated with certainty is that alcoholic drinks will continue to be enjoyed by the majority of adults in the communities in which boys and girls are growing up.

Very little research has been done on the attitudes of boys and girls to drink. But a recent study of the use of alcohol by a sample of boys and girls aged 14–17 years attending schools and colleges of further education in Glasgow (see references) discusses the extent of drinking among them, and attempts to discover possible reasons for adolescent drinking. The analysis suggests that 'toughness' and 'sociability' figure prominently in boys' and girls' perception of drink. These notions are also used, as will be discussed in the following chapter, in investigations into the motivation of children towards smoking, and indeed almost all of the conclusions of this Scottish study indicate a very close parallel with smoking. It would be unwise to generalise from one investigation into the attitudes and behaviour of a group of boys and girls in Glasgow.

Anyone who presumes to offer advice or suggestions to teachers about their approach to the discussion of alcoholic drinks with their pupils is confronted with the immediate difficulty that teachers, like all other adults, vary widely in their own attitudes to drink. Teachers include those to whom total abstinence is the only acceptable way of life, a conviction less common today perhaps, than 50 years ago, but none the less sincerely and tenaciously held; those to whom drinking is an infrequent activity associated with pleasant celebrations and significant social occasions; those to whom regular drinking in moderation is a normal part of life; and a few to whom drink may be a continuous temptation and a refuge. The parents of schoolchildren of course show a similar range of behaviour, with the added complication that among them are members of many races with differing social and religious views on the place, if any, permitted to alcoholic drinks in their lives, and in the lives of their families. So it is tempting to fall back on the advice to tell the children the facts and let them decide for themselves on the basis of the facts—which they are rarely in practice completely free to do— or to tell them nothing.

The first of these alternatives is unsatisfactory because the relevant facts, although important, are not always easy to ascertain. Undoubtedly it is useful for young people to know something of the relative alcoholic strengths of various kinds of drink, the ways in which the rates of absorption of alcohol into the blood stream change with the state of stomach content, and of the forms of loss of control which accompany excessive drinking. And they need to know that if one drink makes them happy 10 drinks will not make them happier. But the chemist's discussion of fermentation and of the properties of ethanol is about as incomplete an explanation of the delights of a fine claret as the biologist's explanation of mammalian reproduction is of the power and passion of mature sexual love.

The second alternative—to tell them nothing—is in practice impossible, as will be realised after a moment's consideration of the difficulties in planning a course of English literature for boys and girls up to 16 years old containing no references of any kind to drinking.

The impracticability of the second alternative may give a key to a more constructive approach. Without regarding alcoholic drinks, or even alcoholism, as yet another matter of social concern demanding emergency shock treatment in schools; without in fact appearing to draw the pupils' attention to the topic, it is easy to think of ways, possibly for application in the primary school but more appropriately with older pupils, in which the subject slips naturally into various parts of the curriculum. Examples are almost obvious. The contribution of chemistry has been mentioned and the contribution of English literature hinted at. The history of England in the 18th and 19th centuries is incomplete without reference to the temperance movements; the trade and geography of Europe incomplete without reference to the wine growing areas; physical education almost certainly includes opportunities to mention the effect of alcoholic drink on physical efficiency; the Old and New Testaments include references to drink; and any discussion of accidents demands facing up to the less attractive aspects of the topic. Home economics may perhaps make the greatest contribution of all, since many civilisations, some near at home, have for generations regarded wine as complementary to food, so the arousal of an intelligent interest and the opening up of the possibility of the cultivation of discriminatory taste in older pupils by discussing the different types of drinks and their compatibility with food may well be the most constructive safeguard against excessive drinking caused by ignorance and bravado. Teachers who include in their work a study of advertisements will find the promotion of drinks a rich field for illustrating modern techniques of mass persuasion, especially interesting to boys and girls, who do not normally like to be 'conned', because many such advertising campaigns are clearly directed at young people and so portray young men and women as enjoying a life style which many growing boys and girls may find highly attractive.

Some heads of secondary schools may not be satisfied that so gradual and piecemeal an approach is sufficient. They may consolidate and deepen understanding among older boys and girls by giving them opportunity to discuss with teachers how to decide their attitudes to drinking. Such discussions will almost certainly include consideration of the reasons why people drink, the dangers of excessive drinking, and guidance on behaviour when in the company of heavily drinking friends. Boys and girls may come to the conclusion that the decision to drink is a personal responsibility, and that even if the decision is taken to enjoy moderate drinking in convivial company, alcohol inescapably remains a drug which must always be treated with respect, since over-indulgence can turn pleasure into misery.

But notions of right and wrong, and the attitudes that do most to determine the behaviour of adults are established at a much earlier age than is often realised. So it is at least probable that by far the most important influence in this, as in other related matters, is the home. The responsibility of parents is fundamental and unavoidable. The schools can only co-operate and, where necessary, supplement—bearing in mind that the misuse of alcohol among adults is far more widespread than the misuse of all the drugs discussed in the previous chapter.

References

Teenage drinking: a cause for concern? (Grassmarket Urban Aid Project Team Report No. 7), R Flint, Edinburgh Grassmarket Urban District), 1974.

'Drinking behaviour in childhood and adolescence: an evaluative review' in *British journal of addiction* vol. 65 pp 203–212, B Stacey and J Davies, Pergamon, 1970.

'Teenagers and alcohol' in *Health bulletin* Vol. 31 (6) 318–319, B Stacey and J Davies, Scottish Home and Health Department, 1973.

Further reading

Notes on alcohol and alcoholism, S. Caruana (Ed.), B Edsall for the Medical Council on Alcoholism, 1972.

Alcoholism, N Kessel and H Walton, Penguin, 1965.

Alcoholism (Report) (enclosure to circulars ML4/73 and ECL 146/73), Standing Medical Advisory Committee for DHSS, HMSO, 1973.

12

SMOKING

Cigarette smoking has recently been described as being probably the most addictive and dependence-producing form of self-administered gratification known to man. Most people who drink do so in moderation: a small minority become alcoholics. But even the most stable well-adjusted person, if he starts to smoke and does not give it up at a very early stage, will become a regular dependent smoker and then find it difficult to stop.

The Royal College of Physicians drew attention in 1962 to the powerful evidence of an association between smoking and lung cancer. In 1971, by publishing *Smoking and health now* they pointed out the strong grounds for the belief that cigarette smoking is not only the prime instigator of lung cancer but a major cause of chronic bronchitis, a significant factor in increasing the risk of illness or death from ischaemic heart disease and other less common conditions, and, if indulged in by pregnant women, a way of increasing the risk of harm to their babies. Recent research points to the probability that the early development of the children of mothers who smoked at least 10 cigarettes a day (especially at the later stages of pregnancy), is relatively both physically and mentally retarded (see references).

Two points need to be stressed before the evidence is reviewed. Cigarettes, if regularly smoked in sufficient numbers, are lethal to some but not to all, and there is a long time-delay between the onset of the habit and resultant death. So this is a matter of probabilities, not of certainties—in contrast with, for example, the certain and rapid effects of a dose of 100 milligrams of nicotine.

The argument rested, in the first instance, on a series of epidemiological studies. It is supported by growing knowledge of the chemistry of tobacco smoke and of its physiological effects, and by experiments on animals.

In 1971, the year of the publication of *Smoking and health now*, sales of cigarettes in the UK fell by about 5 per cent, they then recovered but have been falling since 1973. Since the danger of cigarettes first became a topic of widespread discussion in the early sixties there has been a notable drop in cigarette smoking among men, particularly those in professional occupations. However, there has been little change in the overall proportion of women smoking cigarettes, although in the professional group there has been a marked decline. At the same time the average consumption of cigarette smokers has increased for both men and women—the increase being greatest for young women who are clearly a main target of modern advertising campaigns.

In England and Wales the mortality rate of men from lung cancer rose from 50 per million population in the years 1916–1920 to 869 in 1961, and continued to rise to 1,103 in 1974. In this latter period the rate for women rose proportionately more rapidly, from 139 in 1961 to 261 in 1974. In 1975 more than 26,000 men and 6,750 women died of lung cancer, between a third and a half (or a little over one third) before the age of 65. The proportion of all deaths due to lung cancer is now greatest in men between the ages of 55 and 65, when it is one in every seven deaths, and in women in the age groups 45–54 and 55–64 when it is one in every 16 deaths.

The first attempts to explain the rise in lung cancer were based on statistical studies seeking to establish a correlation between the increase in the disease and changes in behaviour and in the environment. The proportionate increase with time in cigarette smoking and lung cancer gave at least an indication that they might be associated. In the same period there were many changes in the environment: for example, total air pollution increased in the vicinity of country roads because of diesel fumes, yet decreased in the towns because of less smoke from factory and domestic fires as a result of the Clean Air Acts. There were great changes in methods of food production, involving chemical sprays and fertilisers. Industrial developments involving more use of asbestos, chromates, nickel, arsenic and radioactive materials may also have increased the incidence of lung cancer (see Chapter 7 on asbestos). Nonetheless most cigarette smokers inhale smoke, which is thus brought into contact with the lungs, and the rise in consumption of cigarettes made it reasonable to suspect a connection between cigarette smoking and lung cancer.

Epidemiological studies are of two types—retrospective and prospective. Retrospective studies are those in which the previous behaviour and environment of diseased patients are considered. More than 30 such investigations in 10 countries have consistently demonstrated a direct association between the number of cigarettes smoked and the incidence of lung cancer. In prospective studies the behaviour of large numbers of people is recorded throughout their lives so that the factors in their behaviour which may be causes of their deaths or serious illnesses may be ascertained. Such studies obviate some of the bias in retrospective studies which record habits, present and past. after the patient is known to have the disease under investigation. The Royal College of Physicians in *Smoking and health now* gave great weight to five prospective studies carried out in Britain, the United States and Canada.

All of this work points to the conclusion that there is a close correlation between the number of cigarettes smoked (by women and by men) and the chance of death by lung cancer, but none explains why one individual contracts the disease while others with similar smoking habits escape. These investigations also reveal the influence of different smoking habits, the effect of filter tips, the age of starting to smoke and the reduction of risk to those who stop smoking. A survey by E C Hammond (see references) showed that men who began regular smoking before the age of 15 had a death rate from lung cancer five times greater than those who began after the age of 25. The reduction of risk to those who stop smoking was revealed especially in the study of British doctors carried out by R Doll and A B Hill (*Mortality in relation to smoking: ten years' observation of British doctors*—see references). Between 1951 and 1966 half of the doctors included in the study who used to smoke cigarettes had stopped smoking, though over the period there was little change in the general consumption of cigarettes by the population as a whole. Yet between the periods 1953–57 and 1961–65 lung cancer deaths among all men aged 35–64 rose by 7 per cent but fell by 38 per cent among doctors of the same age group. This strongly suggests that stopping cigarette smoking reduces the risk of lung cancer.

The suggestion that a habit which is claimed to bring pleasure to many also greatly increases their prospect of death from an extremely unpleasant disease did not go unchallenged. The argument has been disputed both by questioning the validity of the statistical analysis and by propounding alternative hypotheses. Among the latter are the hypothesis that diesel fumes are a major cause, and a 'genetic' speculation that people with an inherited liability to lung cancer also inherit a desire to smoke cigarettes and that the liability and the desire are therefore related. An unconvincing set of assumptions is required to support these alternative hypotheses as compared with those which support a causal connection between cigarettes and lung cancer. The argument provides a modern example of Occam's Razor.

Epidemiological studies also indicate strongly that smoking is a contributory factor in other illnesses. These include diseases of the lung such as chronic bronchitis and emphysema (an extremely unpleasant chronic condition in which much of the lung has been destroyed by repeated infections, making the patient almost permanently breathless); diseases of the heart and blood vessels; and cancers of the mouth, pharynx, larynx and oesophagus. Some of these conditions are rare, but out of 567,262 recorded deaths in England and Wales in 1971, ischaemic and other forms of heart disease caused 172,000, and bronchitis, emphysema and asthma more than 31,000. There is no suggestion that smoking is the sole cause of these conditions, but a great deal of evidence that it is a significant factor.

Many studies have been directed especially at the effects of smoking on bronchitis and on heart disease. These are discussed in some detail, with references to many research papers, in *Smoking and health now*. The conclusions are summarised in the following two quotations from a report on 'Smoking and Health' by Fletcher and Horn which was presented to the 23rd World Health Assembly in 1970.

'Bronchitis:
Large prospective studies have all shown a steady increase in mortality from bronchitis and emphysema with increasing cigarette consumption, with lower rates in pipe and cigar smokers. In smokers of 20 or more cigarettes a day the mortality is some 15 times greater than in non-smokers.'

'Ischaemic Heart Disease:
Prospective mortality studies agree in showing that mortality from ischaemic heart disease is greater in cigarette smokers than in non-smokers, and increases with increasing cigarette consumption. It is greater in smokers who inhale and in those who started at an early age. This association of cigarette smoking with deaths from ischaemic heart disease is quantitatively different from its association with lung cancer and chronic bronchitis. Ischaemic heart disease is frequent among non-smokers, and the proportionate increase of risk in cigarette smokers is relatively small. It is less directly associated with the number of cigarettes smoked, and the increased risk is greater in younger smokers (two to three times the rate of non-smokers) than in older smokers (50 per cent greater than in non-smokers). Since the disease is so common, however, the small proportionate increase in mortality from it among cigarette smokers results in a much larger total increase in the number of deaths from it among smokers than the total increase of deaths from lung cancer. Pipe and cigar smokers have little or no increased mortality risk as compared with non-smokers. The risk of ischaemic heart disease is increased in people in relation to high blood pressure, obesity, diabetes, raised blood cholesterol loads, physical inactivity, impaired lung function, and personality type. Statistical analyses have shown that cigarette smoking is related to mortality from ischaemic heart disease independently of all these factors.'

The possible effects of smoking during pregnancy on the unborn child have already been mentioned. These effects are, like all the other risks of smoking, certain for some but escaped by others. Growing evidence suggests that smokers' babies are more likely to be aborted, to be still-born or to have congenital heart disease and it has been estimated that in 1970–71, 1,500 babies in England and Wales were lost as a result of their mothers smoking during pregnancy (see references).

A number of papers published more recently have demonstrated the value to health of stopping cigarette smoking; some of these are concerned with single smoking-related diseases and others with general mortality. For example, Reid and others (see references) in a study of coronary heart disease in British civil servants showed that the relative risk of death from this disease was the same in ex-smokers as in never-smokers, and considerably less than in cigarette-smokers, especially heavy cigarette smokers. A study by Doll and Peto (*Mortality in relation to smoking: twenty years' observation of male British doctors*—see references) showed that the overall mortality rate fell among the doctors in the study who had stopped smoking in large numbers, from the fourth to the twentieth year of the study, by 28 pre cent in those under 65 years of age; and by 9 per cent in the same groups among men in England and Wales who as a whole reduced their consumption much less.

There is also recent evidence that smokers who have switched to cigarettes with a lower tar-nicotine yield have somewhat reduced the serious risks of smoking although those who have stopped smoking altogether have fared considerably better (see references—*Some recent findings concerning cigarette smoking*—Hammond and others 1976).

The composition of tobacco smoke, a mixture of gases and minute tarry droplets, is complex (over 1,000 compounds have been identified) and depends to some extent on the type of tobacco plant, the way the leaf is cured and the way it is smoked. The last few puffs contain more tar because it condenses towards the butt end of the cigarette. The substances present may be grouped as:

a. known cancer producers: Carcinogens, which initiate cancer, and co-carcinogens which accelerate cancer formation by the carcinogens.
b. irritants. These may stimulate secretion of mucus in the bronchial tubes and inhibit the action of the cilia (small hairs) which normally sweep out the mucus.
c. nicotine. An alkaloid which acts on the central nervous system.
d. carbon monoxide.

The substances in group a. cause lung cancer when it occurs. Those in group b. play a part in bronchitis and emphysema. Nicotine may stimulate or sedate according to its concentration and to physiological factors in the recipient. The effects of nicotine are fully discussed in various recent papers, and there is growing support for the belief that nicotine is the constituent of tobacco on which smokers rapidly become dependent. Carbon monoxide, when absorbed in the blood, reduces its efficiency as an oxygen carrier and so may increase the possibility of heart disease and be a factor in limiting athletic performance. This latter point has of course been recognised by generations of athletes, but the full significance of the production of carbon monoxide by smokers—both for themselves and for others—has only recently been appreciated. In enclosed spaces such as cars the concentration of carbon monoxide caused by smoking may exceed the level tolerated as safe in industry (see Chapter 6), so that smoking might sometimes be not only unpleasant but also harmful to others.

Many experiments have been performed on animals by making them inhale cigarette smoke, by injecting the condensate of tobacco smoke under the skin or into the lungs of rats, or by painting it on the trachea of dogs. In 1970 it was reported that dogs had developed lung cancer by direct inhalation of cigarette smoke into their lungs, and several experiments had established that condensate can cause cancer when applied to susceptible living cells. The effects of tobacco smoke on the cilia have been studied in the laboratory and in post mortem examinations.

The chemical analysis of tobacco smoke and all the experimental evidence support the conclusions derived from epidemiology.

An expert group appointed by Action on Smoking and Health (ASH), a voluntary organisation whose purpose is to combat smoking, produced a report *Pipe and cigar smoking* in 1973 (see references). They summarised several investigations and concluded that whereas cigarette smokers have between a 50 and 100 per cent greater death rate from all causes at a given age than non-smokers, those who smoke only pipes or cigars are subject to a much smaller increase in risk of death, estimated to range from one per cent to 20 per cent in various studies. Pipe and cigar smokers who smoke moderately and do not inhale have only a very small increase in risk: but the minority who smoke heavily (10 or more cigars or 20 or more pipes daily) and inhale, incur a risk to life similar to that of light cigarette smokers who smoke less than 10 a day. Their risk of dying from bronchitis or emphysema is two or three times greater than that of non-smokers, compared with a ten-fold increase of risk for cigarette smokers. There is little evidence of increased risk of coronary heart disease in light smokers who stick to cigars or pipes, but the chances of developing cancer of the mouth, oesophagus or larynx are increased by all forms of smoking, as markedly for pipe and cigar as for cigarette smokers. The reasons for these differences are believed to be that cigar and pipe tobacco smoke is alkaline and its nicotine content is absorbed through the mouth, while the nicotine in the more acidic cigarette smoke can only enter the blood stream via the lungs—so cigarette smokers have to inhale to get their nicotine whereas most pipe and cigar smokers do not normally inhale. Pipe and cigar tobacco also contains a much smaller proportion of carbon monoxide than cigarette smoke. But animal tests have shown that condensed pipe and cigar smoke is more likely than the condensate from cigarette smoke to produce cancer when applied to the skin, which may account for the incidence in the past of cancer of the lip among habitual smokers of clay pipes.

The accumulated evidence is now such that no reasonable man or woman can deny that smoking increases the risk of both premature death and of severe illness. This is conceded, at least by implication, by the manufacturers of cigarettes who accept that their products should bear a government health warning, who now promote brands of cigarettes by claiming that they are low in tar and/or nicotine yield, and who are searching for safe and acceptable synthetic substitutes for tobacco.

Teachers in many disciplines can, in secondary schools in particular, find ways to contribute to their pupils' understanding of the facts about smoking so that they are better able to make informed decisions. For many years schools have discouraged smoking by their pupils and today there are few secondary schools in which the topic is not discussed at some point in the curriculum. In a growing number of schools smoking by adults is discouraged, and in some it is forbidden. In addition, many primary teachers realise that tentative experiments in smoking are often made by young children in their care so that they have a responsibility to set an example to their pupils. No English curriculum development project in biology has failed to include a factual consideration of smoking (see references) based in the main on the reports of the Royal College of Physicians, while the General Studies (6th form) Project of The Schools Council includes among its publications *Smoking—a scientific study*, in which boys and girls in sixth forms are invited to read extracts from various sources and to draw from them their own conclusions which they must then defend in discussion.

It is sometimes argued that attempts to encourage boys and girls to decide their behaviour in this matter by an assessment of the evidence are unsuccessful, or even futile, because action is determined by attitudes —attitudes of parents or elder brothers and sisters, or friends, or of society. This overlooks the point that attitudes to behaviour are determined by many causes and change gradually but continually. The probability that attitudes to smoking will change as a result of teaching boys and girls to look objectively at and understand the evidence is far greater than the prospect offered by strident campaigns which only invite a hostile reaction from many who believe they are being 'got at' by experts whose reasoning they may only vaguely understand. Change will inevitably be gradual and may be slow, because boys and girls find it difficult, if not impossible, to visualise the possible long-term consequences of smoking; because they know that many older people whom they like and respect, and who may love them, smoke; and also because, as has been suggested earlier, nicotine induces rapid dependence which is very hard to overcome.

During the past decade several attempts have been made by psychologists and sociologists to find out why young people begin to smoke and the extent to which they do so.

The young smoker by J M Bynner (see references) is an interesting and very readable account of a survey which the author undertook in 1966 to find out what attractions smoking holds for children and what pressures are on them to take it up. His evidence suggested that health education may, even in 1966, have had a larger influence than is sometimes admitted and that the health hazard is an inhibiting influence on young boys and girls. He also pointed out that approaches to children have overlooked the fact that most of them smoke so little that the health risk may seem to them to have no relevance, and that the motives behind children's smoking are very different from those of adults who continue the practice, sometimes against their better judgement.

Bynner based his conclusions on a series of tests given to 5,601 boys from each of the first four years (ie in the age range 11–15) in 10 secondary schools during 1966. The questions put to the boys added up to a searching probe into their interests, tastes, attitudes to school, parents and friends, the kinds of people they admired or disliked, their views of boys who smoke, of girls who smoke, of boys and girls who do not smoke, their reasons for smoking, their assessment of their parents' attitude to smoking, and their knowledge of an attitude to the possible dangers of the habit.

There were three main findings:

'First: The main attraction of smoking to schoolboys is the toughness that it represents. Smokers are able to achieve status in the eyes of other boys because smoking symbolises toughness; they therefore have a major incentive for continuing to smoke, and non-smokers similarly have a strong incentive for starting. Smokers are also united with their friends by the value they place on precocity. This gives them an additional incentive to continue smoking because to give it up would mean identifying with non-smokers, a group who appear very immature to them, and who do not value success in attracting girls as they do. The one unattractive aspect of smoking for these boys is its association with lack of educational success. Schoolboy smokers, by and large, want to be successful at school and yet they feel they are failures. Although the main pressure to smoke is probably the need for the smoker to conform with his friends whose interests are in some respects in conflict with school aims, and whose performance at school is consequently poor, many may smoke in order to compensate for their inability to do well at school . . . Smoking as a symbol of identification with achievements in the teenage world outside the school provides an obvious means by which they can achieve status in the classroom.

'Second: The great significance of the extent of parents' permissiveness in the development of the smoking habit. There appear to be a number of conditions in a home which provide the setting for permissiveness towards smoking, and some of these have little direct relation to parents' attitudes towards it. Thus, although parents' own smoking habits seem to be unrelated to their attitudes towards their children's smoking, by bringing cigarettes into the home they increase the availability of cigarettes which itself is one of the preconditions for a permissive atmosphere.

'Third: The considerable success which had been achieved by 1966, when the questions were set, in informing boys of the health risks, in contrast to the relative failure of this information as a deterrent. It was notable that many of the boys expressed concern for the possible effects of smoking on their parents' health, and anxiety because their parents were sometimes unable to give it up. Boys tended to identify the anti-smoking campaign with adult interference and to reject its health message because they resented adults telling them what to do.'

The practical conclusion from this work was summarised by Bynner in the following paragraph:

'The main pressure on a boy to smoke comes from his need to conform with, and gain status in the eyes of, his group of friends. This influence is countered by his parents' disapproval of smoking and by the health risks in smoking. Anti-smoking strategy needs to be directed at devaluing smoking as a means of achieving status in the peer group, at strengthening home restraints, and at increasing the effectiveness of health education.'

Since Bynner's survey was published several similar investigations have been made. Three of them are likely to be of particular interest to teachers.

A small survey by Dr Philippa Poulton (see references) was confined to 331 girls in one grammar school. The girls who smoked, mostly intermittent and light smokers, explained their reasons by phrases such as 'All my friends smoke'; 'I don't want to be left out'; 'I'm afraid to refuse'; 'It's something to do at a party'; 'It relieves tension. I smoke when I'm worrying about exams'; and 'I enjoy it'. She concluded that it is very important that the facts be clearly but undramatically presented, allowing the girls to use their understanding and reach their own conclusions, and that when resentment is aroused by an authoritarian or condemnatory attitude the result may well be a boomerang effect—a conclusion supported by comments from the girls which included: 'I don't like being brain-washed'; 'It's my decision'; 'It's none of their business'. Dr Poulton also drew attention to the need for health education in primary schools because 20 per cent of the girls she interviewed admitted to tentative smoking before they were 11 years old.

Primary school children have been the subjects of two recent surveys by Dr Beulah Bewley and others (see references). The first was planned to discover the prevalence of smoking among a group of children and any correlation between their smoking habits and respiratory symptoms. The summary of their paper was:

'This paper describes the first large-scale prevalence study of smoking by primary school children. Questionnaires on smoking and respiratory symptoms were completed by 7,115 final year primary school children (3,636 boys and 3,479 girls) in Derbyshire. Regular smoking (ie at least one cigarette a week) was reported by 7·9 per cent of boys and 2·6 per cent of girls and a higher proportion of boys experimented with cigarettes. Boys also smoked more cigarettes. Smoking was associated with three reported respiratory symptoms (morning cough; cough during day or night; cough lasting three months or more) and children who smoked more reported more symptoms. Children attending schools in urban areas had significantly more symptoms than those in rural areas. More effective measures to discourage smoking by primary school children are needed.'

The measures referred to in the concluding sentence were not described. Dr Bewley then selected a matched sample of 300 from the 7,115 Derbyshire children included in her first investigation and 293 of them (229 boys and 64 girls) completed a second questionnaire seeking information about their first cigarette, smoking by their parents, siblings and friends, and also their reasons for smoking or not smoking. Because so few girls were included she reported only the results for boys. Not surprisingly only two-thirds of the children were consistent in their replies to the two enquiries.

The replies pointed strongly to the influence of parents and, in particular, of elder brothers and sisters who smoked and lived at home. They also suggested that children rarely buy their first cigarette and gave slight evidence of a peer group among young children. The children were unable to explain why they smoked. Even among the 'heavy' smokers (those who smoked more than one cigarette a day) few said that they enjoyed smoking and a third admitted that their first cigarette had made them sick. Over 80 per cent of boys and girls believed that smoking causes cancer, but many also believed that smoking was not harmful to health—which suggests that some discussion of smoking and cancer is not uncommon in primary schools but that the notion of cancer is (perhaps fortunately) not easily comprehended by young children.

The results of these and other recent investigations do not contradict Bynner's conclusions but suggest a shift of emphasis to the influence of the home, at least in the early stages of smoking, and support the view that the beginnings of health education in this and in many other matters are the joint responsibility of the home and the primary school.

All of these studies, and other recent attempts to classify and to explain patterns of smoking behaviour (see references) indicate strongly that smoking, initially an unpleasant experience, even if attempted only intermittently in company on social occasions rapidly produces a variety of patterns of behaviour whose common factor is dependence on nicotine. Whether this happens is usually settled by the age of 20. McKennell and Thomas (see references) found in 1967 that of those teenagers who smoked more than a single cigarette a day only 15 per cent avoided eventually becoming regular dependent smokers. Whether this happens appears to depend (see references) on the relative weights attached by boys and girls to the following factors:

A. Factors which encourage smoking:
    1. availability of cigarettes;
    2. curiosity;
    3. rebelliousness;
    4. toughness;
    5. anticipation of adulthood;
    6. a lack of social confidence;
    7. parental example;
    8. brothers and sisters smoking;
    9. friends smoking.
B. Factors which discourage smoking:
    1. parental attitude;
    2. school attitude;
    3. health risks;
    4. sensory discomfort;
    5. unpleasant side effects of nicotine.
B4 and B5 decline rapidly as smoking is practised.

Nothing in this analysis weakens the argument for education about health risks. but the analysis suggests that schools could also contribute indirectly to the discouragement of smoking by providing other outlets for some of the encouraging factors in category A. These factors are, of course, relevant only to the beginning of smoking in childhood or early adolescence. Few adults would admit that they smoke because of curiosity, rebelliousness or toughness; some have given up because of health risks. Most continue because of their psychological and physical dependence on the drug nicotine.

This chapter, like chapters 11 and 12, deals with hazards to health about which everyone has to decide for himself. Smoking and all other forms of drug misuse clearly illustrate the processes of modern health education. The first process, the discovery of the facts and estimation of future trends, rests on natural science and on epidemiology. The second and more difficult process is the disentangling of the motives for human behaviour which, in the context of health maintenance, is often irrational. The third process is deciding what educational action, if any, is called for.

In considering how they may help boys and girls to make up their minds about drugs, including drink and tobacco, teachers may find useful a simple analysis of decision-making proposed by M Fishbein (see references). In essence (to simplify further) Fishbein suggests that whenever an individual makes a decision he takes into account:

a. the expectations of others;
b. his personal feelings;
c. his estimate both of the immediate and long-term effects of his decision.

Discussion on these lines with boys and girls can be fruitful. They will soon realise that the expectations of others, such as doctors and cigarette manufacturers, are often in conflict, and may understand why this is so. They will gradually come to see that their personal feelings may be derived from influences of which they are unaware until they are pointed out. They will realise that their estimate of the effects of their decision depends for its validity on the soundness of their knowledge of the matter to be decided.

The influence of the adolescent peer group has been stated or implied in these chapters. The phrase 'peer group' is often used in the literature to explain away behaviour which may puzzle adults, who are usually themselves members of groups of people with interests in common. To suggest that a peer group is not static may be naive, but the point is often overlooked. Any peer group is obviously made up of individual members who are all different. As more join, more share its ethos but they bring their own attitudes, knowledge and beliefs and so they modify the group. Fashions in drugs, in drinking and in smoking, in dress and in many other forms of behaviour change continually. Very few fashions thrive in an adolescent peer group without encouragement by interested adults whom the young may not be aware of—adults who may act in ways they regard as helpful to young people or who may act solely for their own profit. The ultimate responsibility for adolescent peer groups, which may be frivolous, trivial, socially valuable, or extremely dangerous, lies with adults.

References

Smoking and health now, Royal College of Physicians, Pitman Medical, 1971.

The young smoker, Government Social Survey (J M Bynner), HMSO, 1969.

Adults' and adolescents' smoking habits and attitudes, Government Social Survey (A C McKennell and R K Thomas), HMSO, 1968.

'Smoking: Tobacco Dependence', Appendix to Curriculum Paper No. 14 *Health education in schools*, Scottish Education Department, HMSO, 1974.

'Mortality in Relation to Smoking: Ten Years Observation of British Doctors' in *British medical journal* I pp. 1399—1410 and 1460–67, R Doll and A B Hill, BMA, 1964.

Smoking in relation to the death rates of one million men and women (National Cancer Institute Memo. 19, 127), National Cancer Institute, Bethesda, USA (E C Hammond), 1966.

'Smoking and Death Rates' a follow-up of 187, 783 men, in *Journal of American Medical Association* vol. 166, p. 1294, American Medical Association, 1958.

The Dorn study of smoking and mortality among US veterans (National Cancer Institute Memo 19.1.1), National Cancer Institute, Bethesda, USA, 1966.

'Cigarette Smoking Among Grammar School Girls', in *Health education journal* vol. 32 No. 4, Dr P Poulton, Health Education Council, 1973.

Smoking by children in Great Britain, (referred to in *British medical journal* vol. 4, p 3), B R Bewley and others, Research Publications London, 1973.

'Factors Associated with Starting of Cigarette Smoking by Primary School Children', in *British journal of preventive and social medicine* vol. 28, pp 37–44, B R Bewley and others, BMA, 1974.

'Smoking in Pregnancy and Subsequent Child Development', in *British medical journal* vol. 4, pp 573–575, N B Butler and H Goldstein, BMA, 1973.

'Pipe and Cigar Smoking', in *The practitioner* vol. 210, pp 264–267, J D Vince and D Kremer, The Practitioner, May, 1973.

'The Smoking Habit and its Classification', in *The practitioner*, vol. 212, pp 791–800, M A H Russell, The Practitioner, June, 1974.

'The Prediction of Behavioural Intentions in a Choice Situation'' in Modern Psychology Readings, 15: *Attitudes and behaviour*, Ajzan and Fishbein (K Thomas, Ed.), Penguin, 1971.

A national smoking programme (A precis of a report by an advisory committee to the Swedish National Board proposing legislation and other action), Advisory Committee, 1973.

Curriculum Development Material:

Biology teachers' guide III, Nuffield Foundation, Longman/Penguin, 1966.

Biology of man, Section 3 (Secondary Science 3), Nuffield Foundation, Longman, 1971.

Biological science study guide, Sec. 1, Ch. 2, Nuffield Foundation, Penguin, 1970.

Smoking: a scientific study (General Studies Project), Schools Council, Longman/Penguin, 1972.

'Smoking and Health', in *WHO Chronicle*, vol. 24, No. 8, pp 345–370, C M Fletcher and D Horn, WHO, 1970.

'Smoking and other Risk Factors for Coronary Heart Disease in British Civil Servants', in *The lancet*, vol. 2, pp 979–983, D D Reid and others, 1976.

'Mortality in Relation to Smoking: Twenty Years' Observations on Male British Doctors', in *British medical*

journal, vol. 2, pp. 1525–1536, R Doll and R Peto, BMA, 1976.
'Some Recent Findings Concerning Cigarette Smoking' in *World smoking and health*, Vol. 1.1, pp. 40–44, American Cancer Society, 1976.

13

SEX EDUCATION

In 1943 the Board of Education issued a pamphlet entitled *Sex education in schools and youth organisations* (see references). This began with the statement that for some time past there had been a growing sense both of the need to see that children and young persons are suitably introduced to, and properly instructed in, matters of sex and of the responsibility that schools (and youth organisations) have towards securing that such instruction and guidance are given. The writer went on to point out that while accurate and adequate knowledge of sexual physiology, as the mechanism of reproduction, is essential, the most important aspects of sex from the point of view of young people are the emotional and psychological aspects, and urged that towards the end of adolescence there should be instruction and advice directed to the understanding and control of sexual impulse and emotion, leading to the establishment of mutual understanding and respect between the sexes, and, as young manhood or womanhood is approached, to an adequate preparation for marriage.

The significance of this pamphlet was that for the first time an official recognition that schools have a responsibility in this matter was made clear.

Three reports of the Central Advisory Council for Education (England) were published between 1959 and 1967, including the Crowther Report (15 *to* 18) (HMSO, 1959) which discussed changing social needs as a background to its detailed consideration of the education of the 15–18 age range. The report included the following paragraph:

'The problem of sexual ethics is, of course, far wider than marriage. Indeed in the years from 15 to 18 it is not mainly a marriage problem. It seems beyond question that behaviour which would have been rejected a generation ago as improper and anti-social—most people would simply have said wrong—is today tolerated or endorsed by adult public opinion. Young people enjoy a much greater freedom to live their own lives without adult supervision, and to meet and spend their time together as they like without censure and without restraints other than those which their own individual taste or conviction imposes. In this change there has been both gain and loss. It is surely gain that boys and girls, young men and young women, should have the opportunity, which earlier generations often lacked, to get to know one another really well before committing themselves to the choice of a mate. It is surely loss that new guiding rules of behaviour in the changed situation have not been sufficiently developed to replace the old customs which nearly everybody has to some extent abandoned and which some have altogether thrown overboard. Clearly it is not possible for an educational service, which is designed to prepare the young for adult life, to establish by itself such a code. This is the concern of society as a whole, young and old alike. Education can only function within the broad directives of right and wrong which society gives. Teachers and youth leaders are, however, well placed to bring to attention the personal bewilderment and disaster to which this public indecision over moral issues often leads the young. There can be no doubt of the disaster. On 1956 figures, one girl in fifty might expect to give birth to a child conceived before she was 17. It is important to disentangle the two strands—the rise in unsupervised association between teen-age boys and girls; and the virtual disappearance of many of the old rules of right and wrong which were formerly accepted even when they were not obeyed.'

The Newsom Committee Report (*Half our future*) (HMSO, 1963) likewise gave attention to questions of growing up, and succinctly expressed its view in the sentence:

'We are agreed that boys and girls should be offered firm guidance on sexual morality based on chastity before marriage and fidelity within it.'

The members of the Plowden Committee, considering children in their primary schools, reported in 1967 that they had no doubt that children's questions about sex ought to be answered plainly and truthfully whenever they are asked, and added:

'We are unanimous that, if they are able to do it, the proper people to answer children's questions are parents. Young children often find the facts of sexual intercourse incredible. The associate their sexual organs with excretion and that they are also instruments not only of reproduction but of love is difficult for them to believe. When the information is given in the context of a happy home by loving parents it may be more acceptable than if given by someone else, however well intentioned. The fact, however, is that not all homes are happy and some parents still find it embarrassing to discuss the physical details of sex with their children. Who, in such cases, ought to answer the questions and in what circumstances?
'If the parents make their own arrangements there is no problem. If they approach the head teacher of their child's school, he must fit their request into the general pattern . . . Every school must make the arrangements that seem best to it and should have a definite policy, which, in consultation with parents, covers all the children. It is not good enough to leave matters vague and open, hoping for the best.
'So far we have been thinking mainly of the more or less strictly biological aspects of sex, of those which are essentially present in the mating of animals as much as in that of human beings. But human sex involves relationships, and relationships involve ethics; although this side of the matter seldom directly affects primary school children, at least to any depth, it will be there, implicitly, in many of their questions. Direct questions must be answered as honestly as possible, with due regard for parental opinion, but a great deal will

depend on the general human relationships that exist in the school. The foundation for good sexual ethics can be laid in a school in which the children learn to respect and appreciate each other as personalities, to treat everyone with consideration and never to make use of human beings or treat them callously or contemptuously and where they find in adults the same attitude towards each other and towards themselves.'

The handbook of health education (DES, HMSO 1968) naturally reflected and amplified the point of view implicit in these reports of the Central Advisory Council but approached the whole topic of sexual relationships under the heading 'School and the Future Parent', thus emphasising that the production of dependent human beings and the consequent responsibility for their upbringing—not casually to be undertaken—lies at the heart of the matter.

These and other official writings over a period of great change reveal the concern which has been shown about responsible presentation of the problems of sexual development. These comments are so comprehensive as to suggest that no more remains to be said. This is not so because the past decade has seen the growing effects of six factors whose full significance have yet to be evaluated. Perhaps the most important are the growing acceptance of the contraceptive pill and the judgement which allowed the publication of *Lady Chatterley's lover*. The others are changes in the divorce laws making divorce easier; the abortion laws; greater understanding that in a multi-racial society many different attitudes, religious beliefs and social customs exist and must co-exist; and lastly an appreciation that sexuality is a problem for the handicapped which it is now possible to discuss. To some extent these factors are interrelated.

The pill has made it possible for many women to control their fertility with a confidence not previously known and has therefore led to a continuing re-assessment of the role of women in society. It has also encouraged public discussion of the whole field of contraception and family planning related to the problems presented by the growth in the world population. Because the pill is available only on prescription it has also drawn attention to a sensitive area of confidentiality between doctors and patients, especially when the latter are young unmarried girls, possibly still at school. And it may have encouraged the belief that chastity is no longer relevant as a protection against unwanted pregnancy—a belief easily dispelled by a study of the figures for illegitimate births in the past decade. The pill, though useful to the married and to those in stable sexual relationships, is of little value as a guard against the possible consequences of unpremeditated intercourse, because it depends for its effectiveness on a continuous course of medication, which implies premeditation. The Lady Chatterley judgement has led to a decade of freedom of speech, of writing and of action which had not previously been experienced in the United Kingdom by anyone now living; a freedom to which attention is drawn in the cinema, on book-stalls and even by broadcasts in sound and on television. This has been a major factor in the so-called 'permissive society'—a society which may place a burden of decision making in morals and conduct on immature boys and girls at a progressively younger age, and at the same time impose on them strict, exacting demands for self-discipline so that they may equip themselves to earn their living as members of that society. The main point which affects the work of the schools is that they can no longer avoid their responsibilities in sex education because information, often misleading, is thrust at children out of school.

Changes in the divorce laws may have relieved many homes of intolerable tensions, but coupled with the changing status of women they are making the one-parent family more common, so that teachers, especially of young children, need to be very careful indeed when they discuss family relationships. Likewise the presence in society of sub-stantial racial minorities with a range of religious beliefs and of family customs very different from (and often stricter than) those experienced by the majority of teachers imposes a necessity for great caution, toler-ance and understanding. The abortion laws have drawn attention very sharply to an apparently insoluble moral dilemma and it is noticeable that many young people find abortion offensive although they may concede that it is sometimes the least of several evils. Sexuality in the handicapped is being discussed in many countries and the discussion points clearly to a growing acceptance of a variety of sexual practices within certain stable relationships—sometimes marriage—which may have much to do with love but nothing to do with creation.

Fear is sometimes expressed that young people are rapidly becoming increasingly irresponsible in their sexual behaviour. Despite the fall in the average age of menarche—noted for some years but now apparently checked (see references)—the quicker physical development of many boys, the increase in the length of school life, the growth of full-time further education and all the trends in society mentioned in the previous paragraphs, there is little evidence to support this suggestion, at least in boys and girls who are still at school.

Schofield (see references) in a well-known survey (published admit-tedly as long ago as 1965) concluded that sexual intercourse in boys and girls under 18 was by no means universal, and now estimates (*Sex education*—see references) that 34 per cent of boys and 17 per cent of girls are sexually experienced by the age of 18. It appears that although intercourse is a premarital activity of the minority of this age group it is not merely confined to a few.

An investigation into an older age group of girls was published by McCance and Hall in 1972 (see references). In 1971 they surveyed un-married women undergraduates at Aberdeen University with the primary intention of discovering the extent to which they used contraception. They found that 56 per cent of these girls said they were virgins. Thirty-two per cent said they had been sexually active within the six weeks before the survey, and the remaining 12 per cent had had intercourse on earlier occasions. Within the sexually experienced group, six out of seven had a steady boy friend, and over two thirds now used contraceptives. Many admitted that they took risks because intercourse was irregular, infrequent, often unpremeditated, and in different surroundings.

Such statistics take no account of the extent of sexual experimentation short of intercourse practised by young people, and disregard the degree to which sexual activities may be sources of anxiety to boys and girls alike, and may indeed impose upon them conflicts of emotions and of conscience which may be the unsuspected source of stress. Nor do they take into account the explosive nature of sexual behaviour among the young which may impel conduct which gets out of hand more easily than they expect.

The only direct medical indices to sexual intercourse among young people are the notifications of pregnancies and abortions at various ages, which tell us nothing about the fathers, and the statistics for venereal diseases.

The number of illegitimate live births in England and Wales to girls between the ages of 11 and 14 rose from 187 in 1964 to 287 in 1974; to girls aged 15 from 882 to 1,266 in the same period. There were 1,553 such births to all girls below the age of 16 in 1974, and 3,378 legal abortions. So the number of girls below the school-leaving age who were known to be pregnant in 1974 was a little less than 5,000. It is of little comfort to those who have to deal with these girls to reflect that they are a very small minority of the age group. A few may be the victims of rape or incest. Those who work with such girls sometimes report that pregnancy is not necessarily the consequence of ignorance; it may, for instance, be an attempt by the girl to obtain an emotional satisfaction by creating someone whom she believes she will be able to love and who may, for the first time in her experience, love her. Their pathetic state is unlikely to be relieved by giving them more effective knowledge of methods of birth control but, if this diagnosis of the cause of their action is correct, it can only point to a failure of home and school to offer them opportunities to establish bonds of communication, friendship and status with their peers and experience the taste of achievement, however modest. Several local education authorities have issued advice to schools confronted with pregnancies among the girls. The annual totals of illegitimate live births in England and Wales are shown overleaf in Table IX.

The incidence of gonorrhoea has risen in England and Wales from a minimum of 20,000 new cases in 1955 to about 59,000 by 1975. Most cases occur in the age range of 16–24, with a very sharp increase in

HE—H

rate from 5 per 100,000 population under the age of 16, to 302 per 100,000 in the 16–17 age range, to 665 in the 18–19 group, with 600 in the 20–24 range. Likewise cases of other genital infections, which are not necessarily due to changes in sexual partners, rose rapidly in England from 70,000 in 1951 to 300,000 in 1975. The possibility of gonorrhoea among school children is remote, but below the age of 18 girls are about two and half times as likely to contact the disease as boys, presumable as a result of intercourse with older men. The incidence of gonorrhoea points to the activities of a relatively small number of promiscuous young men and women. Probably many of the women have symptomless infections of which they are unaware.

Table IX
Illegitimate live births in England and Wales

Table X
Abortions to single women (residents in England and Wales)

Year	Number (000's)	Year	Number (000's)	Year	Number (000's)
1945	63·4	1966	67·1	1968	10·3**
1955	31·1	1967	69·9	1969	22·3
		1968	69·8	1970	34·5
		1969	67·0	1971	44·3
1960	42·7	1970	64·7	1972	51·1
1961	48·5	1971	65·7	1973	52·9
1962	55·4	1972	62·5	1974	53·3
1963	59·1	1973	58·1	1975	52·4*
1964	63·3	1974	65·5		
1965	66·2	1975	54·9		

*notifications
**for the period 27 April—31 December 1968

The decline in the number of illegitimate live births since 1967 should be seen in relation to the statistics for abortions in single women shown in Table X.

These facts show how far the religious ideal of chastity is from universal acceptance. Although, as has been pointed out earlier, it is at least doubtful if wider knowledge of methods of birth control would significantly reduce pregnancies among girls below the school leaving age, the argument for making such knowledge (or at least the sources of such knowledge) and/or professional help available to older boys and girls, before they leave school, seems difficult to contest.

'Education in personal relationships' is an implicit function of all communities, including all schools, and in the still controversial field of sex education there is a growing consensus that whatever the phrase 'sex education' may mean it is certainly inextricably bound up with the physical, emotional and mental development of children, especially in adolescence, and for many with their not too far distant prospect of parenthood.

In the majority of schools a great deal of consideration is given to the role the school should play in preparing boys and girls to cope with problems which demand of them decisions about their behaviour, now and in the future. In other words they have to evolve a considered basis of morality, of which sexual conduct forms only a part, but a part of such importance that it may lead them to a sacramental relationship of profound significance, or, at the other extreme, to the broken home, ruined children's lives, or destroyed careers so they may ask in despair:

'What win I if I gain the thing I seek?
A dream, a breath, a froth of fleeting joy.
Who buys a minute's mirth to wail a week?
Or sells eternity to get a toy?
For one sweet grape who will the vine destroy?'
The rape of Lucrece.

The question to be decided in every school is the extent to which the school, in co-operation with parents, has a responsibility in helping boys and girls to arrive at moral decisions which involve understanding of relationships essentially sexual. There is no practical possibility of avoiding the issue, as was illustrated by a school in which the headmaster declared that there was no sex education in his school, while the English specialists in the sixth form were reading and discussing in depth John Donne's love poetry in lessons in which the master superbly illustrated Wilson's judgement (*Practical methods of moral education*—see references), that:

'Any teacher worth his salt will be too interested in helping the pupils to make up their own minds to be seriously worried by his own "commitments". For that is what education is about. Provided he has a prior commitment to reason, truth and charity which over-rides his own particular beliefs— and if he has not then he should not be a teacher—he has no need to trouble himself unduly over this problem.'

This is a high ideal. In practice, it may be necessary to raise further questions about objectives and methods.

Those who embark on a deliberate policy of sex education and education in personal relationships in schools of all types are faced with the following questions:

1. Why? What are the aims, both short-term and long-term? This is the most difficult question of all but it must be answered before going on to:
2. Who should be responsible for the teaching? Many boys and girls are embarrassed by 'trendy' teachers, and all are immediately aware of hypocrisy and dishonesty in adults, and many teachers are embarrassed by the task.

3. What underlying value judgements are assumed? These must be identified and defended.
4. What are we going to teach? A foundation of biological knowledge? If so, will it include information about family planning, contraception, venereal diseases, and sexual deviations?
5. At what stages in school life will the teaching be attempted, and why?
6. What methods of teaching will be adopted? Exposition, discussion, individual counselling, individualised learning (tapes, projected material, books etc for private study)?
7. To what extent are the influences of the whole curriculum and the life of the school taken into account? This is a very important question because discussion of sexual matters can so easily be over-emphasised.
8. How does the school co-operate with parents and others responsible for the children?

There are no standard answers to these questions applicable to all types of school. A great deal of discussion of them is to be found in the reports of several working parties set up by local authorities, which tend increasingly to consider such matters as part of their suggestions for health education in the context of social education. Discussion and helpful suggestions, especially for teachers in secondary schools, are also included in several recent curriculum projects, including Nuffield Biology, Nuffield Combined Science, Nuffield Secondary Science (Theme 3), and the Schools Council's Moral Education, Humanities, and General Studies projects whose contributions have been summarised by Dorothy Dallas (see references).

The Churches and other interested bodies have issued discussion papers. The BBC and Independent Television continue to produce a range of broadcasts planned to help teachers responsible for various age groups. The following miscellaneous comments may perhaps also help in considering some of the questions involved.

The growth of understanding is very gradual, and attempts to pass on knowledge have to be related carefully to particular stages of a child's development which are not accurately indicated by age. Most parents and teachers probably agree that boys and girls should be prepared for the bodily changes of puberty, especially for natural (and possibly disturbing) processes like menstruation and nocturnal emissions. It is wise that these changes should be understood by both boys and girls. Boys in particular should come to realise that for girls there are times connected with menstrual periods or with episodes in their emotional development when they may be distressed or tired through no fault of their own, and that both should realise that the emission of semen is abundant, and sometimes uncontrollable. Girls should also understand that they may quite inadvertently impose great stresses on boys by arousing sexual reactions in them which they do not fully comprehend and may not be able to control. As integrity and respect for truth are basic in this, as in all teaching, it is dishonest and futile to hide, at the proper time, that sexual intercourse should be highly enjoyable—if this were not so most of this chapter would not have to be written—and that it includes much more complex activities than elementary accounts of reproduction suggest. The growth of understanding of this, with all the associated issues of sexuality, of love, of the powerful and sometimes overwhelming emotional involvements of men and women, is necessarily very gradual, and if approached clumsily before boys and girls are mature enough to begin to comprehend is likely to do more harm than good. One of the reasons for imparting basic knowledge of reproduction is to allay anxieties which may arise from fantasies based on ignorance, or from feelings of inadequacy. The very greatest care must be observed not to set up even more damaging anxieties in boys and girls who still prefer their hobbies and interests while some of their contemporaries are blatantly attracted to the opposite sex, by implying that they are not developing normally and so making them feel themselves forced into patterns of precocious experimentation which are an affront to their innate sense of modesty and decency. It is vitally important that the privacy and reticence of boys and girls are respected by teachers, and that teachers should never in any circumstances lift the veil from their own private lives.

Masturbation, which used to be called self abuse, is now regarded as an inevitable but transient part of developing sexual awareness. This innocuous practice may start in infancy and continue until maturity is reached. Only when masturbation occurs in public should notice be taken as it may then be an indication of disturbance which could need psychiatric treatment.

Contraception is likely to be heard of by quite young children. Although the methods are very easily understood in general terms, once the outlines of the reproductive process have been grasped it is important to discuss with pupils the morality and purposes of contraception, including the important factor of the growth of regard for the quality of life and of responsibility for others. Saying 'no'—probably by far the most widely used method of avoiding unwanted pregnancy by young girls—is also by far the most certain. A knowledge of contraceptive methods, whether by creating physical and chemical barriers, or by interfering with the monthly cycle, or by choosing times in the cycle when fertilisation is least probable does not of itself assure their use. The most effective way of dealing with the techniques of contraception is to make certain that all boys and girls understand and have confidence in the professional services available to them as they grow up.

The venereal diseases need some consideration in secondary schools, for again they are the subject of public discussion of which older boys and girls are usually well aware, and they may already be of practical concern to a few of them. It is advisable to explain that they are a direct consequence of sexual intercourse, including homosexual practices, and that anyone suspecting infection has an inescapable duty to seek cure and to help in tracing contacts. The diseases are described in Appendix 1.

Sexual deviations should not be mentioned unless specific questions are asked, as they may be. Teachers universally accept that they have a duty to warn children never to accept lifts or sweets from strangers, without necessarily spelling out the dangers from which they are protecting them (whether of a sexual nature or otherwise).

Homosexuality, both male and female, is probably best dealt with in passing if and when it arises, as it may with older boys and girls from their studies of literature, visits to the theatre and cinema, and from television programmes. Questions, when asked, can no more be brushed off than can the young child's questions about where babies come from. But it is unwise to embark on speculations on the complex and imperfectly understood causes of these relationships, and it is essential to allay fears among boys and girls that close friendships with members of their own sex suggest that they are incapable of heterosexual relationships.

The quotation from the Plowden report at the beginning of this chapter draws attention to the role of the parents of young children in sex education. Few will dispute that parents of children of all ages have the chief responsibility but this does not absolve the schools. This is an area of teaching in which co-operation between parents and schools is not only essential but often highly effective in encouraging mutual understanding and trust. Teachers are wise to give parents opportunity to examine and discuss with them innovatory courses of sex education or personal relationships. Parents are wise to realise that schools can neither avoid references to the broader issues by other boys and girls nor confine the mention of sexual matters to a programme of sex education. Parents may sometimes be disturbed by reports of aspects of sex education and wish to withdraw their children from the lessons: but they may pause to reflect that if they do their children will certainly ask their friends what happened when they were excluded, and will almost certainly receive a garbled report.

Throughout this discussion of the sexual element in education for personal relationships emphasis has been given to the thought that the most important judgement demanded of teachers is to decide for each pupil the appropriate time at which various topics may be broached without doing more harm than good. This is of course true of all teaching, with the difference that in the teaching of, say, physics, if the timing is wrong the worst that can follow is incomprehension or boredom, but in this uniquely personal and individual field the consequences of such misjudgement may cause anxiety which is much more serious.

The final point is that the subject matter of this chapter deals with but one aspect of the process of struggling towards maturity which occupies the first two decades of life; essentially a process of establishing self identity. Teachers and parents alike may usefully ponder the implications of E M Erikson's remark (see references):

'Like a trapeze artist the young person in the middle of vigorous motion must let go of his safe hold on childhood and reach out for a firm grasp on adulthood, depending for a breathless interval on a relatedness between the past and future and on the reliability of those he must let go of, and those who will receive him.'

References

Sex education in schools and youth organi-, *sations*, Board of Education, HMSO 1943 (out of print).

'Changing Social Needs', Ch. 4 in *15 to 18* (The Crowther Report), Ministry of Education/Central Advisory Council for Education (England), HMSO, 1959.

'Spiritual and Moral Development', Ch. 7 in *Half our future*, (The Newsom Report), Ministry of Education/Central Advisory Council for Education (England), HMSO, 1963.

'Aspects of the Curriculum' Ch. 17 in *Children in their primary schools*, (The Plowden Report), Ministry of Education/Central Advisory Council for Education (England), HMSO, 1967.

'End of the Trend?' A twelve-year study of the age of menarche, in *British medical journal*, vol. 3, pp 265–267, T C Dann and D F Roberts, BMA, 1973.

'Sexual Behaviour and Contraceptive Practice of Unmarried Female Undergraduates at Aberdeen University' in *British medical journal*, vol. 2, pp 694–700, C McCance and D J Hall, BMA, 1972.

The rape of Lucrece, W Shakespeare, lines 211–215.

The Sexual behaviour of young people, M Schofield, Longman, 1965.

Practical methods of moral education, J Wilson, Heinemann, 1972.

Sex education in school and society, D M Dallas, NFER, 1972.

Insight and responsibility: lectures on the ethical implications of psychoanalytic insight, E M Erikson, Faber and Faber, 1964.

Further reading

Sex education: rationale and reaction, R Rogers (Ed.), CUP, 1974.

Sex education in perspective: a symposium on work in progress, National Marriage Guidance Council, 1972.

The sexual behaviour of young adults, M Schofield, Allen Lane, 1973.

14

MENTAL HEALTH

However health is defined mental health is an important, if not the most important, element, and it is reasonable to ask if programmes of health education in schools can contribute to mental health in adult life, or (to turn the question round) do anything to lessen the prospect of a period in a mental hospital which now confronts one in nine men and one in six women in England and Wales. This question is not to be confused with asking what parents and schools can do to reduce the number of disturbed pupils, although the answers to both questions are related. This second question has been touched on in Chapter 11.

In 1975 the Secretary of State for Social Services presented to Parliament 'Better Services for the Mentally Ill'. Its introductory paragraphs contain a helpful description of the nature and classification of mental illness.

'*Mental illness and mental health*
1.1 Mental illness (and conversely mental health) is notoriously difficult to define. There is now a deep interest in the psychological aspects of human behaviour, collectively as well as individually; an interest which is constantly extending to new facets of everyday life in society. There is growing recognition of the relationship between behaviour and environment; and indeed there are probably few aspects of public and private activity that have not been held to have some effect, whether direct or indirect, on our psychological well-being. At the individual level there is an increasing readiness to seek counselling, or other forms of professional psychiatric help over an ever wider range of personal psychological problems. As our knowledge and awareness of the inter-relationship between physical, emotional, social and environmental factors increases so no doubt this process will continue; more people will seek help and the boundary of what we collectively regard as mental ill-health will be set further back. Indeed we must recognise that the potential demand for psychiatric help is virtually unlimited*. We must ask ourselves to what extent such demands are realistic: not only in terms of finance and manpower, for manpower constraints will inevitably impose their own limits, but also in as much as they represent unreal expectations of what psychiatric help can do.

'1.2 Changes in the nature of the problems for which individuals consider they need psychiatric help imperceptibly change society's general concept of what is mental illness and what is not; how far behaviour can be regarded as eccentricity and a reflection of individual personality; how far behaviour calls

---

*As long ago as 1966 a research study suggested the presence in all communities surveyed of a large sub-group of emotionally sick or emotionally disturbed patients amounting to between 1/5 and 1/10 of the total population.

for punishment and how far for treatment. But we should beware of over-emphasising this, particularly in the context of current psychiatric practice in this country. It is new advances in scientific knowledge and understanding that have enabled, for example, the sufferings of the housebound phobic or the young girl starving herself through anorexia nervosa to be recognised for what they are—namely the manifestation of mental illnesses for which it is both humane and realistic to offer professional help.

'1.3 How do we then define mental illness? On the one hand "mental illness" as a term probably still has a certain stigma attached to it and most of us probably draw our own fine dividing line between the more comprehensible and respectable forms of mental ill health and the more frightening or distressing forms which we privately label as mental illness. But on this kind of definition the mentally ill would constitute only a small proportion—in practice mainly those with psychotic illness—of the total numbers of those who are currently seeking and receiving help from general practitioners and psychiatrists for psychological problems of various kinds, from severe depression, and phobias, through a whole range of sexual, marital and other human relationship problems. Equally we have to acknowledge that there are many problems of human behaviour—often causing great distress—for which psychiatry can offer little or no remedy and for which other forms of help and support may be more relevant. Attempted suicide is often a case in point. In recent years the numbers of attempted suicides have risen sharply. Research suggests that only a minority of those concerned suffer from psychiatric illness as such; but often there is a background of longstanding personality and relationship difficulties.

'Is mental illness increasing?
1.4 The difficulties involved in measuring the prevalence of mental illness and in particular in making comparisons between prevalence rates in different places and at different points in time will be immediately apparent. The point has already been made both that to some extent society is constantly redefining its concept of mental ill-health, and that advances in scientific knowledge enable us to understand and treat mental suffering which, insofar as it was previously untreatable, was in the past not regarded as illness. These two processes go hand in hand. Surveys of prevalence based on the number of contacts made with relevant health and social services will only reflect the extent to which people in practice seek professional help for their psychiatric or psychological problems. Conversely as and when new treatments are developed and facilities are both readily available and accessible they will themselves call forth new demands. Morbidity surveys run up against the difficulty that they are liable to reflect individual researchers' concepts of mental illness.

'1.5 We are tending to widen our definition and our recognition of psychological distress. But is the underlying incidence of such distress also increasing? Are we in fact living in a society which is positively giving rise to mental ill-health? There is no hard evidence to confirm that the incidence of mental illness is increasing but undoubtedly there are features of modern industrial society which many people feel make them more vulnerable to mental stress: high-rise flats for families with young children; production line work with no job satisfaction; the break-up of the large family unit; overcrowded living conditions; the pressures of advertising with its suggestions of "norms" of happiness, friendship and sexual satisfaction and the consequent feelings of inadequacy among those who have not achieved them.

'Estimates of prevalence
1.6 The second National Morbidity Survey carried out in 1970–71 by the Office of Population Censuses and Surveys surveyed 53 general practices in England and Wales serving some 300,000 people, and found that on average over the year 1 in 14 males and 1 in 7 females consulted their general practitioner for some form of mental illness. This would be equivalent to about 5 million people nationally. However, several recent surveys have suggested that general practitioners themselves may not always detect psychiatric symptoms—or recognise them as such—and there is little doubt that much mental illness, some of it serious, goes undiagnosed and untreated. True need is almost certainly much greater than present demand. The proportion of those who consult their general practitioner who are referred to the specialist services is about 12 per cent. It has been estimated that about 600,000 people nationally receive specialist psychiatric services each year. This estimate is based on information from psychiatric case registers which have been established in some parts of England and Scotland and in which all contacts with specialist services from a given population are recorded. But numbers, however great, cannot measure the sum of human misery, the tragic waste to the community of creative talents, drive and enthusiasm and, the bitter disruption of family life and relationships which mental illness often brings.

'Classification by diagnostic group
1.7 Over recent decades there has been much debate both within and between different professional groups about the nature and classification of mental illness. The increased involvement of a widening range of professions—psychologists, social workers, sociologists, geneticists and biochemists—has led to the recognition of new dimensions of the problem and new theories. What is, perhaps, most encouraging and, indeed, impressive, given the enormous scope of the problem, is that in recent years widespread research has led to a growing consensus of opinion among the different disciplines that mental illness is not the result of any single factor but is caused by a wide range of factors, social, familial, and genetic, and is similarly multi-faceted in its manifestation. Classification is not easy: there is often overlap between some of the generally accepted disgnostic groupings and the severity of symptoms for the same disgnosis varies from one individual to another. Such problems are, however, found in all branches of medicine to varying degrees and are by no means confined to psychiatry. Similarly, as in other fields, a clinical diagnosis by itself will often be of limited significance in determining certain of the patient's needs. But in the field of mental illness there can on occasion be a real danger in giving a patient a diagnostic lable, particularly where this is liable to follow him throughout his life and place him on the wrong side of the dividing line between public acceptance and understanding, and public rejection and fear.

'1.8 Classification is, however, important. It is the starting point for much comparative research, for investigating the causation of identified patterns of psychiatric disturbance, and it is through informed debate that further knowledge and understanding will be gained. While, therefore, in the following paragraphs mental illness is described on the basis of the Mental Disorders section of the International Classification of Diseases, this is done in full recognition of the limitations of any one approach.

'*The neuroses*

1.9 The principal distinction normally drawn is that between the psychoses and the neuroses. The sufferer from neurotic illness retains his consciousness of the real world about him but certain of his behaviour patterns become exaggerated by fears or depression to such an extent that they interfere with his normal daily life. People with neurotic conditions account probably for more than one-third of all referrals to psychiatric services. Depression and anxiety or tension states are perhaps the most common. The OPCS survey found that during 1970–71 20 males per 1,000 and 47 females per 1,000 attended general practice with a diagnosis of anxiety neurosis. The corresponding figures for depressive neurosis were 15 and 47 per 1,000. Depression and anxiety states will vary greatly in degree, in some cases being no more than a relatively short-lived response, perhaps, to bereavement or a new situation, in others severe and prolonged and with no obvious external cause. It should be emphasised that the prevalence of these conditions is much greater than that of psychotic illness.

'*The psychoses*

1.10 The sufferer from psychotic illness, as the condition advances, is distinguished by his tendency to lose contact with his surroundings and his distorted view of the world around him. The largest single group of psychoses are those known as schizophrenia or the schizophrenias. The onset of schizophrenia, perhaps the most disabling of all forms of mental illness, occurs generally in the teens to early adulthood with hospital admission rates being highest among the 25–34 age group. The prevalence rate for adults, in terms of numbers of people in contact with the specialist psychiatric services in any one year, is approximately 1 in 300. Schizophrenia is often accompanied by a withdrawal into a world of fantasy and auditory hallucinations, with disturbance of volition or drive, and as it progresses there may be accompanying physical deterioration. A variant may start with the onset of delusions of persecution. Another group of psychoses, known as affective psychoses, has been estimated as having a comparable prevalence rate of about 1 in 280. They tend to occur later in life and are characterised by changes of mood that cannot be accounted for by external causes alone. The schizophrenias and the affective psychoses are together included in a group of mental illnesses known as the functional psychoses. Though no single theory of causation has yet been established it is possible that they have an inherited biochemical basis, but are precipitated by environmental factors. There is a clearer understanding of the physical basis of a further group, known as the organic psychoses. Acute confusional states may be reversible depending on the associated physical condition. Dementia on the other hand, seen mainly in the elderly, is the result of the death of some brain cells and leads to intellectual deterioration and lack of emotional control and drive. It is an irreversible and generally progressive process, the prevalence of which has been shown to increase greatly among persons in their late seventies and eighties.

'Psychopathic disorder
1.11 The Mental Health Act 1959 defined psychopathic disorder as "a persistent disorder or disability of the mind (whether or not including sub-normality of intelligence) which results in abnormally aggressive or seriously irresponsible conduct on the part of the patient and requires or is susceptible to medical treatment". The term "psychopath" has come to carry a considerable stigma and there has been a reaction against it in favour of "personality disorder with antisocial trends" since this is thought to convey a better idea of the range of problems involved. Personality disorders affect people of a wide intelligence range, and seem to be inherent personality traits rather than illnesses as such. Those with personality disorders have in some cases an apparent lack of ordinary appreciation for the feelings of others, and a common characteristic is an inability to learn by experience. They are often considered as having an immaturity of personality which may manifest itself in many different ways: at one end of the spectrum they may be highly disruptive members of society and commit serious crimes. At the other it may result in no more than an inability to organise a settled life, often with a consequent tragic descent down the social scale. The individual's basic difficulty in coming to terms with society may, however, manifest itself in many ways, each in some way an attempt to resolve his apparently insoluble problems.

'1.12 There is considerable uncertainty about the extent to which people with personality disorders can be helped by the mental health services and there is undoubtedly a need for further research and new approaches in this field. It is generally accepted that such people do not readily respond to traditional psychiatric treatment and indeed there are difficulties of principle in determining those cases in which it is proper to regard a behaviour pattern as a "disorder". Nonetheless in recent years there has been a sharp increase in the number of admissions to hospital for personality and behaviour disorders. People with serious personality disorders not infrequently become involved with the police. They also present considerable problems for social services departments. There has recently been much debate as to whether, and if so to what extent, it is appropriate for them to be admitted compulsorily to psychiatric hospitals. The present position is that the concept of susceptibility to medical treatment is applied to compulsory admission; and this has led to difficulties in certain areas in the placement of psychopaths appearing before the Courts. The question of psychopaths who offend against the law has been studied by the Committee on Mentally Abnormal Offenders, chaired by Lord Butler, which has recently completed its report.'

' Distinction between mental illness and mental handicap
1.14 Mental illness is quite distinct from mental handicap. Mental handicap is usually determined before or during birth or in the early weeks of life and is characterised by intellectual retardation which affects the ability to learn and reason. It maybe accompanied by physical and psychiatric handicaps. Though the development of the mentally handicapped person can be improved by training, education and social care, mental handicap cannot be cured and is a lifelong condition. Mental illness, however, can occur at any age and affects people of every intellectual level. (Some mentally handicapped people also suffer from

mental illness.) While in the present state of medical knowledge by no means all forms of mental illness can be completely relieved, advances over the last 20 years mean that most functional illness will now respond to treatment.'

Many neuroses—and especially the symptoms acute anxiety and depression—are attributed to stress. Stress, like mental health, is in this context very difficult to define but the physician's definition of stress as the observable consequence of a strain may not entirely beg the question, because a strain is a set of forces. Any physical material which is stressed will return to its original state when the strain is removed unless the strain exceeds a limit characteristic of the material, when the material will be permanently deformed. This, in physics, is said to happen when the elastic limit of the material is exceeded. The analogy goes quite a long way when applied to human beings who are strained. The forces which strain them may be many, such as bereavement, loneliness, exacting and prolonged demands on skill and energy, the pain of personal conflict culminating in a broken marriage or in a prodigal son, a too rapid change of environment from, for example, the dirt and friendliness of the slum street to the sterile isolation of the high rise flat, or even what a distinguished Oxford don once described as the initial fate of freshmen (and sometimes the fate of boys and girls joining a secondary school), the loneliness of the crowd. Other strains may have been applied in the past, long before the stress manifests itself, by parents or by forgotten incidents in early life. Stress may, and often does, result in purposeful action, but sometimes the elastic limit is exceeded. Stress is an essential ingredient in any creative human activity, as was suggested by the anonymous writer who implied that the discontented philosopher was mentally healthier than the contented pig. Stress, as an ingredient in creativity in men and women of genius, sometimes manifests itself in various forms of behaviour which many would regard as eccentric, if not outrageous. Newton, Florence Nightingale, and Tchaikovsky will serve as examples; the reader may think of many others. The problem in school, as in life, is to get the degree of stress right for each individual at different stages of development.

The contribution to mental stability which health education at school can make is very largely that of giving boys and girls some insight into these complex matters so that they will react to cases of mental illness with sympathy and understanding, and come to appreciate how great is the responsibility of everyone not to aggravate stress by cruelty (of which they may not be fully aware) or lack of consideration for others. Although they may realise that adults often appear to prefer conflict to co-operation, human societies have evolved methods of ameliorating abrasive contacts, known as codes of courtesy or good manners.

Another contribution comes from the growing involvement of boys and girls in voluntary work for the welfare of others, especially the old and the mentally handicapped. This encourages understanding and may lead to helpful discussion. The reader may care to answer the following questions, posed recently to boys and girls in a course in health education in a mixed secondary school, and to estimate the extent to which such discussion, based on observation and knowledge, may be constructive.

1. Would you be worried at the thought of having to go into a mental hospital for treatment? If so, why?
2. Have you ever visited a patient in a mental hospital? What was it like and what sort of treatment was the patient having?
3. Do you feel sympathy for people who have nervous illnesses, or do you think they should 'pull themselves together'?
4. Why do you think people are encouraged to paint, write and read poetry, or to do handicrafts when they are getting better from a nervous illness?
5. Do you know any subnormal people? How do you feel about them?
6. Do you think it a good idea to try to train them to help themselves? How do you think the community should treat them?

The merit of such an indirect approach, with adolescents, to the simpler ideas of mental functioning is that it enables the teacher to avoid the risk of insensitivity towards conflicts which may be troubling them.

References

Curriculum planning and some current health problems (Education Studies and Documents No. 13), (W H Southworth), UNESCO, 1974.

Mental illness and mental health in the world today, M G Candeau, WHO, 1969.

'The Extent of Mental Illness in England and Wales' in *Health trends*, vol. 6, No. 3, pp 56–59, DHSS (E R Bransby), HMSO, 1974.

Better services for the mentally ill, DHSS, HMSO, 1975.

Further reading

'Mental Health: a Physiological Model', in *Community health*, vol. 6, pp 286–291, A J Dalzell-Ward, 1975.

'Mental Health', Chapter 11 in *A textbook of health education*, A. J. Dalzell-Ward, Tavistock Publications, 1974.

Appendix 1

NOTES ON SOME COMMON COMMUNICABLE DISEASES

Diagnosis of disease and prescription for its treatment are medical responsibilities, and for teachers to attempt either would be both unwise and dangerous. But teachers are particularly well placed for co-operating with school doctors and nurses. They may be able to recognise the signs of illness at an early stage, ensure that advice is sought in good time, and help to see that such advice is carried out. Every teacher should have some knowledge of the common communicable diseases and their characteristic features.

Measles
Measles is a highly infectious disease among young children caused by a virus which is spread by droplet infection. It presents as a febrile catarrhal illness affecting the upper respiratory tract and eyes, and resembles a common cold. A rash appears on the fourth day, first around the face and neck and spreading over the body: the illness subsides within three or four days. Mortality is greatest among young (under two years) or debilitated children; it is frequently associated with complications affecting lungs, ears, kidneys, and heart, and these may lead to chronic ill-health or permanent defects such as deafness. Measles frequently occur in epidemics in unprotected populations.

Effective vaccines to control measles have been available for about 10 years.

Mumps
Mumps is caused by a virus which produces inflammation and swelling of the salivary glands. These glands are situated in the floor of the mouth and in the cheeks in front of the ears, causing the patient to have a moon-faced appearance when affected by this disease. It is spread by droplet infection and produces fever, with pain and tenderness of the swollen glands. It is normally a mild illness which subsides in a few days, but it may occasionally be complicated by involvement of testes or ovaries especially in those who are over the age of puberty, which may result in sterility. A high degree of immunity follows an attack.

Chicken Pox
This is a highly contagious febrile illness frequently found in children. It is caused by a virus, which may be spread by droplet infection or by direct contact with an infected person. The condition is mild and begins

with a blotchy rash of the skin which quickly proceeds to watery blisters which then dry to form crusts. It is no longer considered necessary for all scabs to have disappeared from the skin before a child may return to school, and exclusion for six days from the first appearance of the rash is sufficient.

German Measles (Rubella)

German measles is a febrile illness caused by a virus; it is characterised by a rash on face and trunk which may resemble that seen in measles or scarlatina. It is a mild disease causing some enlargement of the lymphatic glands in the neck. There are no complications for the patient, but the rubella virus may have a disastrous effect on the foetus if the disease is contracted by a pregnant woman in the first four months of her pregnancy. The virus may attack and cause permanent damage to developing organs in the foetus, which is then born with often untreatable defects. In babies, defects of eye-sight and hearing, cardiac abnormalities and severe retardation may occur either singly or in combination. Pupils who develop German measles should not return to school until they have recovered and in any case not until four days have passed after the onset of the rash. Female members of school staff who have not had the disease, and who are in the early stages of pregnancy, should be advised not to attend school during an outbreak of this disease until the period of infection has passed. Because of the risk of foetal abnormalities schoolgirls at about the age of 13 are nowadays being immunised against rubella.

Scarlet Fever

Scarlet fever is caused by a haemolytic streptococcus and is spread by droplet infection from infected cases or healthy carriers who harbour the streptococci in their noses or throats. The incubation period is short (two or three days) and the onset is sudden, with fever, sore throat, headache and vomiting, with the appearance of a bright red rash within 24–48 hours. The condition responds rapidly to antibiotics. Although there has been a continuing decline in the incidence and virulence of scarlet fever, it still remains one of the common infections among school children.

Diphtheria

Diphtheria is a highly infectious disease caused by a bacterium which produces lesions in the throat or nose, and more rarely on the skin. It is spread by droplet infection from an infected person or from a healthy carrier. It is a particularly serious condition, especially in young children, and it may be complicated by obstruction of the windpipe, cardiac failure and paralysis of muscles. In unprotected communities the disease reaches epidemic proportions with a high rate of complications and death. The incubation period is short (one to five days) and the illness begins with what appears to be an ordinary sore throat, rapidly followed by the appearance of a grey-white membrane covering the back of the throat, and signs of prostration. Diphtheria immunisation is given to children in the first year of life as the greatest incidence of mortality and morbidity is among infants. The full course of immunisation requires that three doses be given at intervals, and these are usually given combined with whooping cough and tetanus vaccines; a booster dose should be given at the age of entry to infant school. Diphtheria immunisation is an excellent example to justify the adage that prevention is better than cure; as noted elsewhere there has been a dramatic fall in the prevalence of this disease because of widespread immunisation. But the acceptance rates for immunisation must be kept up, or isolated cases of diphtheria will occur among unprotected children.

Tuberculosis
Tuberculosis in man is caused by the tubercle bacillus and is spread by droplet infection. The bacillus causing human disease is either the human or the bovine strain, the latter being a common cause of the disease in cattle, which may contaminate milk from an infected udder. This bacillus has high powers of resistance to bacteriocidal agents and can survive for long periods if not exposed to direct sunlight. The droplets from an infected person or particles of dust and fluff contaminated by the bacillus are inhaled into the lungs and produce a primary reaction which has an innate tendency to heal, producing a degree of immunity to the disease. This immunity, however, may be overcome by poor general health, by overwork, by fatigue, by overcrowded conditions, and by association with repeated doses of infection from an open (sputum positive) case of the disease resulting in the appearance of disease in the patient. Tuberculosis attacks almost all the organs of the body, but is most frequently seen as pulmonary tuberculosis; usually it is a chronic disease leading to progressive destruction of lung tissue.

Bovine tuberculosis attacks lymphatic glands and bone but this form of the disease has been less commonly encountered since the practice of pasteurisation of milk was introduced which eradicates the bovine strain of the tubercle bacillus. The prevalence of all forms of tuberculosis has been steadily declining in this country over the past few decades. This has been due to a variety of factors such as improved conditions in housing and places of work, improved economic conditions, programmes for BCG vaccination, contact tracing and supervision, and new drugs which reduce the natural reservoir of infection.

Whooping Cough (Pertussis)
Whooping cough is a highly infectious disease of young children and is caused by a virus. It is spread by droplet infection. The onset is

gradual and indefinite, and the disease presents as a catarrhal illness of the upper respiratory tract with a gradual appearance of paroxysmal coughing and characteristic whoop. Uncomplicated whooping cough terminates equally gradually so that it is often difficult to recognise that the disease has ended. Whooping cough immunisation gives protection against the disease and is frequently given in association with diphtheria and tetanus immunisation in the first year of life.

Food Poisoning

Outbreaks of food poisoning due to bacteria or bacterial toxins may occur in schools. Food acts as a culture medium for the growth of food poisoning bacteria which comprise three main groups. Most frequently involved are the salmonellae, next are the clostridium welchii and more rarely the staphylococci. The onset of the symptoms of food poisoning may be as short as two to three hours after eating food, or as long as 36 hours. Usually a number of people who have eaten the same food are affected and the illness is mild with nausea, vomiting, diarrhoea and abdominal pain. However, the staphylococci can produce an enterotoxin which produces more severe symptoms, including collapse and prostration; these symptoms usually occur within six hours of eating the contaminated food. High standards of personal hygiene in both kitchen and teaching staff and among school children are essential in avoiding outbreaks of food poisoning; known carriers of disease should not be involved in handling food.

Poliomyelitis

Poliomyelitis is a virus infection which may occur sporadically or in epidemics; it is spread by close contact with an infected person. The virus is present in the pharynx for a week after infection, but may be excreted in the faeces for periods of three to four months. Strict control of hygiene arrangements in schools will help prevent spread of this disease which is highly infectious in young children particularly in unprotected communities. The incubation period may vary from three to 21 days, but commonly is two to three weeks. Poliomyelitis may present as an illness characterised by malaise, lassitude, tiredness, vomiting, mild headache, sore throat or slight feverishness. In many cases the disease is aborted at this stage, but in others, after an apparent recovery period of three or four days, the disease manifests itself by the appearance of a flaccid paralysis of the affected muscles.

The prevalence of poliomyelitis in this country has decreased dramatically since the introduction of vaccination on a national scale some 20 years ago. Oral vaccine is now offered to all children in infancy, the basic course consisting of three doses (beginning at six months, with second dose six to eight weeks later and third dose at the age of 12–14 months). It is recommended that reinforcing booster doses be given on entry to school and at the age of 15 to 19 years. Children who develop acute poliomyelitis should be excluded from school until they recover; home contacts should be revaccinated and excluded from school for three weeks.

Sexually Transmitted Diseases

The incidence of sexually transmitted diseases (venereal diseases) has been increasing steadily over the last 10 years in all parts of the world, including England and Wales where there has been a sharp rise in the number of cases of gonorrhoea. A medical reason for this increase in sexually transmitted diseases is that some of the organisms causing these diseases have been found to be increasingly resistant to penicillin and other antibiotics.

Sexually transmitted diseases are spread by close sexual contact with the body of someone already infected. The organisms live in the sexual organs and die very quickly away from the heat of the body, therefore it is practically impossible to catch these diseases from lavatory seats, towels, bedclothes, door handles or dirty cups. More than half the women infected have neither signs nor symptoms of the diseases and do not know they are infected. They are a reservoir for venereal diseases.

There are about 15 conditions which can be spread from one person to another by sexual contact. Some are serious, others are minor skin complaints that cause inconvenience and tend to reduce the quality of life but do not affect general health. The conditions include syphilis, gonorrhoea, non-specific urethritis, trichomoniasis, candidosis, herpes genitalis, chancroid, lymphogranuloma venereum, genital warts, scabies, pediculosis pubis, molluscum contagiosum, balanitis, tinea cruris, and vaginitis.

Gonorrhoea is the commonest form of sexually transmitted disease and is caused by the bacterium *Neisseria gonorrhoeae*. The incubation period is from two to ten days after intercourse but may be rather longer in females of whom 35 per cent with gonorrhoea have no symptoms at all, but are carriers of the disease. Gonorrhoea in men causes inflammation of the urethra which produces a burning sensation on passing urine and a yellow or green discharge from the tip of the penis. This condition is so painful that it cannot be missed.

In women the discharge produced by the infection can pass unnoticed as it mingles with the normal secretions from the vagina. Occasionally there is frequency in passing urine accompanied by a burning sensation but such symptoms can occur after intercourse in women who are not infected by gonorrhoea. If untreated, gonorrhoea may spread to other parts of the body causing general ill-health, swollen joints and sterility. A baby born to a mother who has gonorrhoea can have its eyes infected by the germ, and unless treated this infection can cause blindness.

Syphilis is a far less common venereal disease but it is extremely serious and affects men and women in the same way. It is caused by the spirochaete *Treponema pallidum*. Ten to ninety days after intercourse with an infected person a painless ulcer (chancre) appears on or near the genitalia or any part of the body that has been in contact with the infection. The ulcer is highly infective and a woman may not realise that one has developed in her vagina and so may inadvertently continue to spread the disease. The ulcer will disappear of its own accord but without treatment the germs will spread throughout the whole body. Some weeks later the second stage of the disease develops with a rash, fever, sore throat, and sometimes loss of hair. These signs will also disappear without treatment but the germs will remain in the body and infect every organ. There then comes a latent stage that can last from six months to 40 years when syphilis can only be diagnosed from blood tests, often made for other reasons. Routine blood testing at ante-natal clinics has led to the treatment of expectant mothers and the reduction in the incidence of congenital syphilis. After the latent stage tertiary syphilis develops. This can mimic other diseases and may eventually cause paralysis, blindness, insanity and death. In a pregnant woman suffering from syphilis the germ will pass through the placenta and affect the foetus. The baby can be born dead or diseased, with permanent physical and mental defects.

Non-specific urethritis is a venereal disease whose incidence has increased considerably in men and now exceeds that of gonorrhoea. It is a milder disease than gonorrhoea; the incubation period is seven to twenty-eight days, and although women are thought to be carriers they are symptomless. The organism responsible may be a virus-like agent (chlamydia) or a mycoplasma. The infection causes a discharge from the tip of the penis which can last for months. Occasionally unpleasant complications such as prostatitis, or a condition where the eyes and joints are affected, known as Reiter's disease, occur. It is rather difficult to cure. Treatment with the antibiotic tetracycline clears the condition but it tends to recur and can present a considerable problem.

Even though the organisms responsible for gonorrhoea, syphilis and non-specific urethritis are developing resistance to some antibiotics, nearly everyone who contracts a venereal disease can be cured if treated in the early stages. In England and Wales there are 200 special clinics diagnosing and treating sexually transmitted diseases. They are attached to major district hospitals and by telephoning one of these the telephone number of the special clinic can be obtained and through this an appointment can be made. Treatment is by suitable doses of penicillin but as the resistance of some of the organisms develops larger and multiple doses of penicillin, sometimes combined with other expensive antibiotics, have to be used. Syphilis needs a longer period of treatment but can be cured in the first two stages, but if the tertiary stage is reached damage already done by the disease cannot be repaired. As some women do not have symptoms, contact tracing by specially trained social workers is one of the most important ways of controlling the sexually transmitted diseases, since there is no known means of conferring immunity.

Communicable Skin Diseases

Verminous Conditions

The prevalence of head lice among school children fell slowly after the last war until the mid-sixties when a gradual increase was noted. The reservoirs of verminous infestation are with the 'problem' families often living in slum conditions, though through the school contacts of a child even the cleanest of families may become infested. While the aim of the school nurse is to provide treatment for the child and the family, this may only be accomplished by full co-operation by the members of the family: regrettably in these problem families such co-operation is not always forthcoming. Evidence of resistance of head lice to DDT and dieldrin insecticides has been steadily accumulating over the past decade; and this has, no doubt, contributed to the rise in prevalence. The emergence of the resistant louse, aptly named 'super louse', has led to the search for newer insecticides, one of which, malathion, has an egg-killing action as well as being very lethal to the louse.

Infestation in schools spreads quickly unless the condition is controlled by regular inspection and treatment. The school nurse advises parents of the verminous child as to the treatment required to eradicate the head lice, and follows up to ensure that the child is free from vermin. The LEA have powers provided in the Education Act 1944 to cleanse the verminous pupil, exclude him from school or prosecute the parent. Regular inspection of the hair and a maintained regime of personal hygiene are important to prevent infestation. Cleansing and the use of a fine steel comb will be required to remove these parasites and their eggs from the hair of an infected pupil.

Impetigo

This contagious skin disease is caused by streptococcal or staphylococcal infection which may be spread in a variety of ways from a septic lesion either by direct or indirect contact with an infected person. It may be a secondary complication of other skin conditions such as scabies, ringworm or verminous infestation. Impetigo begins as thin-walled blisters which are ruptured by scratching as they are very itchy: scratching may also result in the transmission of the disease to other parts of the skin. The most common areas affected are the face and ears and the condition often attacks children. The lesions are usually circular and vary in size: if untreated they heal spontaneously in four to six weeks. The condition quickly responds to antibiotics. Strict personal hygiene and cleanliness will prevent spread of the disease.

Scabies

Scabies is an inflammation of the skin caused by the itch mite (*Sarcoptes scabiei: hominis*). The mite burrows into the skin but the symptom of intense irritation does not appear until several weeks after the first infestation. The itching is due to a sensitisation reaction in the patient and scratching causes the secondary infection commonly associated with scabies. The rash produced by the mite may take several forms but the commonest is the appearance of thin sinuous burrows around the wrists and between the fingers. Treatment, which should be intensive, is highly effective. All home contacts should be treated at the same time.

Ringworm Infections

Ringworm is due to a fungus infection of the skin and is transmitted from an infected person or animal (including cattle, dogs, cats and horses). The condition is due to a superficial infection of the skin which digests the dead horny layer: living skin tissue is rarely involved. Ringworm of the scalp is almost entirely confined to children below the age of puberty and appears as circular lesions with fragmentation and shedding of the hair. The onset is gradual and if untreated the condition may spread to involve eyelids and neck. Most common is ringworm of the feet (athlete's foot) which occurs in the young and middle aged and may be seen in schools in adolescents; it appears as an itchy weeping lesion starting in the clefts between the toes. In severe cases it may spread to the nails and legs. Ringworm responds readily to modern fungicides. Care and attention should be given to personal hygiene and clothing during an attack.

Warts

Common warts are caused by a virus infection of the skin. They may be single or multiple and are most often seen on the hands but may also occur on the face, arms, legs or scalp. Children and adolescents are most frequently susceptible to them. Warts are lesions of about 1·5 mm diameter which protrude from the skin and have a rough horny surface. They are transmitted by direct contact and the incubation period may vary from one to six months.

Plantar Warts

Plantar warts are also caused by a virus infection and are found on the soles of the feet. Unlike warts on other parts of the body they grow inwards so they remain undetected until symptoms such as pain on walking develop. They occur in school children, especially those of secondary school age, and girls are more often affected than boys. The condition is spread by barefoot activities, especially in swimming baths and showers where wet skin is abraded on rough surfaces, so distributing the virus. Prevention is important because plantar warts can be extremely painful and are sometimes difficult to treat.

The necessary measures for this include regular foot inspections, avoidance of communal use of socks and footwear, regular cleaning (with disinfectants) of floor surfaces used during barefoot activities, and the use of disinfectant in footbaths. Infected pupils who take part in activities in which the other children are barefoot should wear plasticised socks. Pupils with plantar warts should wear shoes which are exclusively theirs.

Reference: *Prevention of plantar warts by the use of protective footwear in swimming pools.* Mary H Bunney. Community Medicine, page 127, 1972.

Appendix 2

NOTES ON SOME COMMON PHYSICAL DEFECTS

a. Children's eyesight

The child's eye will usually have reached its full size by the fourteenth year, but slow growth may continue in some individuals up to the age of 23, when the general growth of the human body is usually complete. It seems unlikely that the growth of the eye can be influenced by any factor other than nutrition, which affects the eye like any other part of the body. Infants are usually long-sighted, but this long-sightedness decreases during childhood. Binocular vision, which makes possible accurate fixation and perception of distance, develops slowly up to the age of 6 or 7.

The need to look after their eyesight throughout life should be impressed upon children by training in good habits. Schools should ensure that as much natural light as possible gets into classrooms and that adequate artificial light is provided when required. Direct sunlight can cause difficulties, and blinds may be needed. When children are writing the light should come from the left, unless they are left-handed, when of course it should come from the right; in any event strong cross-shadows should be avoided. School books should be printed in a clear and reasonably sized type and children should be warned against reading badly printed books at home. Glare from polished surfaces can cause fatigue. It is dangerous to look straight at the sun. Reading in bed will do no harm if the light is good, so long as the reader sits up with his book held evenly in front of his eyes. Television viewing is so extensive in homes and its use has increased so much in schools that children should be told about the best posture and conditions for viewing. They should be comfortably seated with the TV set at a convenient level, distance and position for good all-round visibility so that they do not crane their necks, and the room should not be darkened. In this country, the ultraviolet light rays in natural daylight are never strong enough to do the eyes any harm.

Children should be encouraged to mention any difficulty in seeing what is written on the blackboard or in a book. They should realise that if glasses have been prescribed it is to their advantage to wear them at the times advised; teachers should encourage children to follow this advice. Defective vision is sometimes a cause of educational retardation. Frowning, blinking, the rubbing of eyes, the book held too close to the eye, and headaches may be early signs of defective vision. All pupils suspected of having a visual defect must be referred to the school doctor or nurse.

Normally the tears keep the eye protected by washing away germs and dirt, so that the daily use of expensive eye lotions is quite unnecessary. For occasional bathing of the eyes, a pinch of salt in a few tablespoonfuls of boiled water will serve well. Children should learn never to rub an inflamed eye, and that any rag or towel used to bathe or wipe their eyes should not be used by anyone else.

Sight should be examined at regular intervals from infancy. As soon as any squint is noticed, treatment should be started; otherwise the child may fail to use the squinting eye properly, and efficient binocular vision may never develop. Children just learning to read may suffer from strain on their muscles of accommodation, which can be relieved by the temporary wearing of glasses until their eyes are fully grown. The eye lengthens as it grows, particularly during the growth spurt at puberty, so that the development of short-sightedness is common at this stage.

b. Hearing
It is dangerous to put any foreign body into the ear, and a blow on the ear may lead to serious harm; all children should be made aware of this. Sometimes children are troubled by wax. The formation of wax is a normal process, though some people get wax in the outer ear more quickly than others; if the wax accumulates, it should be removed only by a doctor or nurse. The Eustachian tube, which connects the ear with the throat, is much shorter, wider, and straighter in the child than in the adult, and this may have something to do with the greater number of ear infections in young children as compared with adults. Every child should be taught always to blow his nose gently, either without closing the nostrils, or gently closing one at a time, so that there is no risk of transferring nose and throat infections up the Eustachian tube to the middle ear. Since discharge from ears can often lead to impaired hearing, its seriousness should be emphasised and parents should be encouraged to see that children suffering from ear infections receive early, regular, and persistent treatment. Swimming must not be allowed while a child has a cold in the head or a discharging ear. The ears should always be washed carefully, preferably with a washcloth wrung out so that too much water is not allowed in.

Defects of hearing which should be referred to the school doctor are usually less obvious than defects of vision. Hearing may be deteriorating for some time before it is noticed; a child's apparent inattentiveness may sometimes be a sign of unsuspected bad hearing. An upper respiratory tract infection can cause temporary deafness and a child who appears to have intermittent hearing loss should be referred for examination.

c. Care of the feet
In children flat feet without any other abnormality of the lower limbs rarely needs treatment or special exercises.

That the feet should sweat is only natural, although some individuals have trouble with feet which sweat too much. The feet should be washed every day and then dried thoroughly, especially between the toes; socks or stockings should be changed as often as necessary. Like shoes they should be of the correct size to allow for foot growth.

Foot troubles are the cause of much discomfort and inefficiency among adults, especially women. Although foot defects have for years been the object of observation and study there is still not complete agreement on the primary cause. Many claim that the basic cause is an inherent weakness of the foot itself; others maintain that apart from congenital defects and the results of injury, foot deformities are due entirely to unsuitable footwear, particular during youth. It has long been recognised, too, that foot deformities can be found in those who have always worn good footwear and also among those who have always gone unshod. Nevertheless it is reasonable to assume, and there is supporting evidence, that the two important factors are foot strength and suitability of footwear, both of which can be influenced. A child's foot is a mobile, growing structure that adapts itself to the shape of the shoe it is wearing; if shoes are badly designed and their fit is poor, the feet may in time become deformed but it is surprising how seldom children complain of pain, even when their feet are very deformed. It is also regrettable that there is a time lag between the trauma and the defect becoming obvious. Children's feet can stand a great deal of ill-treatment. Those with strong feet are probably able to wear bad shoes for varying periods without apparent ill effect, whereas those with weak feet need good shoes which help to support their poor muscles. There can be no excuses for such common practices as buying shoes by post without a proper fitting or handing them down to younger brothers or sisters as older children outgrow them. Well shaped shoes should be available in half-sizes and a range of width-fittings. If children are to grow up having healthy feet, the state of their shoes and socks is most important. Shoes should be waterproof, strong and well-fitting; they should be pliable yet firm enough to give proper support, so that the foot can develop without cramping or distortion. Most of the fashionable women's shoes are not suitable for growing girls. Many of the fashions are modified for child wear but such shoes should only be worn for short periods. Wellingtons are excellent in wet weather, but these and light rubber-soled shoes (of plimsoll type) should not be worn for long periods. It is inadvisable for children to change into plimsolls on arrival at school and to remain in them all day. Girls as well as boys should be provided with thick boots or shoes for field games such as hockey.

For children and adults alike, shoes and socks are usually needed during working hours. Yet no one who has watched a baby kicking, crawling or learning to walk will fail to realise how good it is for the human foot to have opportunity of moving free and unencumbered by any trappings. Most adults find that the conditions of civilised life make this impossible, except when bathing, or playing on the sand, or performing special exercises; but for children, and especially young children, there should be more scope. Not that they ought to play everywhere in bare feet; the possibilities vary according to climate, place and circumstances, and in many places the risk of cuts from glass, nails or sharp stones would make shoes always necessary. But, particularly in infant and junior schools, there is much to be said for providing the children with opportunities for play or general movement in bare feet during the physical education periods.

See also the notes on ringworm infections (athlete's foot) and on plantar warts in Appendix 1.

Appendix 3

RESOURCES

The emphasis on individual inquiry in schools mentioned in Chapter 1 implies the need for adequate resource materials in the form of books, pamphlets, newspaper cuttings, photographs, posters, wall charts and manuscript materials as well as audio-visual devices which include slides, film strips, films, tapes and video-tapes. In all these respects health education is liberally served by a growing volume of material for all ages, so large that selectivity is the real problem for the teacher.

The mother of the pre-school child may have been influenced by posters on display at pre-and post-natal clinics dealing with cleanliness and food hygiene, and by other simple charts. Many of these could with advantage be used in infant schools to supplement much of the normal play equipment—such as the shop, Wendy house, cleaning sets for mopping, dusting and sweeping—which a teacher might use to emphasise and establish sound health practices. The use of posters, particularly on road, fire and water safety, models, cut-out figures, flannelgraphs and well-illustrated books all help to foster the development of health education.

A great deal of health education is undertaken incidentally in junior schools through project work which requires the collecting and organisation of resource material. At this stage too, the observation and care of animals is often encouraged, and science, which sometimes involves observations of themselves, is begun by the boys and girls. Two cautions are necessary. The care and handling of animals is an important branch of applied hygiene, not to be undertaken without the necessary knowledge. Advice is included in *Safety in science laboratories*, DES Safety Series No 2 (HMSO) and teachers are urged to read *Keeping animals in schools—a handbook for teachers*, (HMSO). The other caution, which applies with even more force in secondary schools, relates to experiments on pupils. This merits the inclusion here of the following quotation from *Safety in science laboratories* paragraphs 128, 130 and 131:

'128 Experiments using pupils as the subject of experiment raise a number of special problems. Before any such experiments involving procedures which are outside the range of normal every-day experience are conducted, teachers should ensure that the pupils understand fully the precautions to be taken and the possible consequences of not taking them. There must be no pressure on the pupils to perform the experiment. The approval of the School Medical Officer of Health should be sought in all cases which involve the tasting of any substance other than foodstuffs and simple chemicals which are known to be safe in the quantities used. No chemical should be swallowed. Similar approval should also be obtained before proceeding with any experiment which involves unusual ventilation of the lungs, unusual physical stress, or any surgical operation, however minor as; for example, in blood sampling with its attendant risk of the transmission of infective hepatitis if sterile procedure cannot be guaranteed. Experiments involving unusual ventilation of the lungs can be dangerous to epileptics, asthmatics, and children who suffer from a wide range of bronchial conditions which may not be known to the teacher or to the child. Teachers may also find it advisable to obtain the prior consent of parents for such experiments. Because, however, it is likely to be difficult to establish that a pupil undertook the experiment in full knowledge of the possible hazards, and with his or her full consent, teachers may consider it advisable to avoid all such experiments with pupils under 16.

130. Under no circumstances should any experiments be conducted or demonstrated in which chemical means (ie drugs) or physical means (such as electrical stimuli) are used in an attempt to affect the mental state of a subject.
131. It has been reported that experiments have been conducted in a few schools on the use of the electroencephalogram (EEG) in so-called biological feedback. Teachers are strongly advised that they should neither perform such experiments nor in any way encourage self-experimentation by their pupils.'

Other human resources (as advisers to teachers or as speakers to pupils) referred to in this pamphlet include (among others) doctors, health education officers, health visitors, nurses, the police, and road safety officers.

Responsibility for co-ordinating and encouraging health education in the secondary school includes responsibility for discovering and assembling adequate resources. These include knowledge of appropriate broadcasts, direct or indirect references to health education in many curriculum development programmes, and the services by way of information and advice offered by a variety of voluntary organisations. The increasingly prominent role played by the BBC and by Independent Television is especially valuable to many schools, both in the quality of their programmes and in the references and suggestions for further work in their booklets.

Fortunately for teachers the Health Education Council has established at its headquarters (78 New Oxford Street, London WC1A 1AH) a national library of resources and will advise teachers on their selection. Many health education officers regard knowledge of this field as of great importance. The range of information may perhaps be illustrated by the references in this pamphlet, which include such diverse sources as the Registrar General's Statistical Reviews, the World Health Organisation, the Department of Employment, the Open University, and reports from Scotland, Australia, United States and Canada.

The Health Education Council publishes very useful source lists (publications and teaching aids) in all fields of health education, with the caveat that these "do not purport to be exhaustive and inclusion does not imply recommendation by the Council". Other bodies publish similar lists covering their special interests. Health education officers in many authorities prepare lists of suggestions and most, if not all, of the reports of LEA working parties on health education include suggestions for further reading. The Health Education Council is able to inform teachers of the activities and addresses of many voluntary societies concerned with various aspects of health education. The references which follow include a list of relevant curriculum development projects—published or in preparation. This list does not purport to be exhaustive, and of course the Department of Education and Science has neither the wish nor the right to imply recommendation.

References

Safety in science laboratories (Safety Series No. 2), DES, HMSO, 1976 2nd edition.

Keeping animals in schools a handbook for teachers, DES, HMSO, 1971.

Source lists:

Health Education Council,
Sex education,
Nutrition,
Food hygiene,
Smoking and Health,
Alcohol Education,
Dental Health

Curriculum development material

Combined science 11–13 *years*, Nuffield Foundation, Longman/Penguin, 1970.

Secondary science 13–16 *years* (Especially Theme 3), Nuffield Foundation, Longmans, 1971.

O-level biology 11–16 *years*, Nuffield Foundation, Longmans, 1966.

A-level biological science, Nuffield Foundation, Penguin, 1971.

Sciences 5–13 Project Ourselves: a unit for teachers, Schools Council, Macdonald Educational, 1973.

Food Science and Technology, Schools Council Project Technology, Heinemann Educational, 1973.

'Patterns 3—Energy' *Integrated Science* in *Project*, Schools Council, Longman/ Penguin, 1974.

Moral education in the secondary school, Schools Council, Longman, 1972.

The family, Schools Council, Heinemann Educational, 1972.

Relations between the sexes, Schools Council, Heinemann Educational, 1972.

General Studies, Penguin Education, 1972.

Schools Council project: Health education (5–13), Thomas Nelson, 1977.

Health education project, in preparation, Health Educational Council.

Printed in England for Her Majesty's Stationery Office
by McCorquodale Printers Ltd., London

HM 7895   Dd 586795   K160   7/77   McC 3309